ACKNOWLEDGMENTS

I express my deepest gratitude to Professor Dr. Stephen H. Curry, chairman of my supervisory committee, for his invaluable guidance during my graduate career and the course of this research project. I am also grateful to him for accepting me and providing me with training support and facilities after Dr. Garrett's retirement.

My very special thanks go to Professor Dr. Edward R. Garrett for his guidance and patience for more than three years. I am very grateful for the moral support and for the sound scientific education he provided me and also for the personal kindness he showed me during my troubled time in 1986.

I also wish to thank the members of my supervisory committee, especially Professor Dr. Alistair Webb whose assistance, skill and knowledge made these studies possible.

I gratefully acknowledge the financial assistance provided by the College of Pharmacy and the Palestine Student Fund for providing me funds for more than ten years.

Special thanks go to Mrs Patricia Khan for all her help and kindness during the past six years and specially in the preparation of this dissertation. Dr. Gina Aeschbacher and Mr. John Bliss should not be forgotten because his skill in handling the animals and assistance in performing the studies were invaluable in the success of this project.

My deepest thanks go to Dr Jurgen Venitz for all his advice, friendship and moral support for the past four years.

Last but not least, my sincerest thanks to Miss Jaimini Patel for her friendship and kind company and support during the last four years of my studies.

TABLE OF CONTENTS

LIST OF TABLES

x

List of Figures page

Abstract of Dissertation Presented to the Graduate School of
the University of Florida in Partial Fulfillment of the
Requirements for the Degree of Doctor of Philosophy

PHARMACOKINETIC STUDIES OF ACEPROMAZINE IN THE HORSE AND THE
CAT STUDIES IN LIPOPHILICITY, RED BLOOD CELL PARTITIONING AND
PROTEIN BINDING

By

Patrick J Marroum

August 1990

Chairman: Dr. Stephen Curry
Major Department: Pharmaceutics

The pharmacokinetics of acepromazine were investigated
in the horse and the cat. The overall objectives of this work
were 1) to study the physicochemical characteristics of six
clinically relevant phenothiazines; 2) to study the
pharmacokinetics and pharmacodynamics of acepromazine in the
horse; and 3) to study the bioavailability of acepromazine in
the cat after oral, subcutaneous and intramuscular
administration.

The various compounds were assayed by means of an HPLC
system with electrochemical detection developed specifically
for this research. Partition coefficients were measured
between hexane and phosphate buffer (pH 7.4), between red
blood cells and plasma and between red blood cells and
phosphate buffer (pH 7.4). Studies in horses involved

intravenous doses, collection of frequent blood samples and assay of the acepromazine content of these samples. The pharmacodynamic measurements consisted of measuring the hematocrit, blood pressure, heart rate, blood gases and the sedative effects of the drug. Studies in cats involved intravenous, oral, subcutaneous and intramuscular doses, collection of frequent blood samples and assay of them for their drug content as well as measurement of the hematocrit. The bioavailabilty of acepromazine in the cat was determined for all the administered routes.

After intravenous administration, acepromazine followed biphasic pharmacokinetics in both the cat and the horse. In general, the pharmacodynamic effects of acepromazine persisted much longer than detectable plasma concentrations of the drug. Acepromazine markedly decreased the hematocrit in both animal species tested. Additionally, there was a decrease in the blood pressure and a marked sedation in the horse after an intravenous dose of 0.15 mg/kg. Intravenous and subcutaneous doses gave concentrations much higher than oral doses. In two cats, intamuscular doses gave plasma concentrations higher than subcutaneous doses. It seems likely that oral doses of acepromazine undergo a very high first pass effect as observed with other related compounds in humans.

There was no concentration dependency for the red blood cell partitioning between phosphate buffer (pH 7.4) and the red cells. Additionally, there was no relationship between the lipophilicity of the phenothiazines studied as measured by their hexane- phosphate buffer (pH 7.4) partition coefficient and the extent of the red blood cell partitioning.

CHAPTER 1

INTRODUCTION

The use of drugs for the treatment of psychiatric disorders has become widespread since the mid-1950s. Today, 20% of the prescriptions written in the US are for medications intended to change the mood or behavior. Phenothiazines, which are major tranquilizers or neuroleptics, are mainly used to treat psychosis. Classification of these drugs can be on the basis of chemistry (e.g. benzodiazepines, phenothiazines, tricyclic antidepressants), neuropharmacology (e.g., neuroleptics, amine re-uptake inhibitors, GABA antagonists) or use (major tranquilizers, minor tranquilizers, antidepressants). One particular phenothiazine (acepromazine) is used only in animals as a sedative preanesthetic drug.

The specific objective of this research was to describe the pharmacokinetic properties of acepromazine in certain domestic animal species. A method of analysis using high pressure liquid chromatography (HPLC) with electrochemical detection was developed. Other relevant pharmacokinetic properties such as red blood cell partitioning and plasma protein binding were investigated.

1

In addition, because of the significance of the physicochemical properties of drugs in drug disposition, an investigation of the relationship between lipophilicity and RBC partitioning was undertaken.

Historical Background

The first phenothiazine was synthesized by Bersthen in 1883 while synthesizing dyes related to methylene blue (1). However, it was until the late 1940s that a derivative of phenothiazine promethazine was found to have antihistaminic and strong sedative properties. Also in that period, Gilman, Shirly, and Charpentier independently synthesized a series of 10-dialkylaminoalkyl derivatives which had weak anthelmintic, trypanocidal and antimalarial properties. In 1951, Charpentier and coworkers, while investigating the central nervous system action of phenothiazines, were successful in synthesizing chlorpromazine (2). Courvoisier in 1953 described the many pharmacological actions of chlorpromazine (3) and Laborit reported that chlorpromazine potentiated anaesthesia and induced a state of artificial hibernation consisting of hypothermia, decreased metabolism and reduced oxygen requirements in patients (4).

The basic phenothiazine nucleus is tricyclic, two benzene rings are attached to each other by a nitrogen and a sulfur

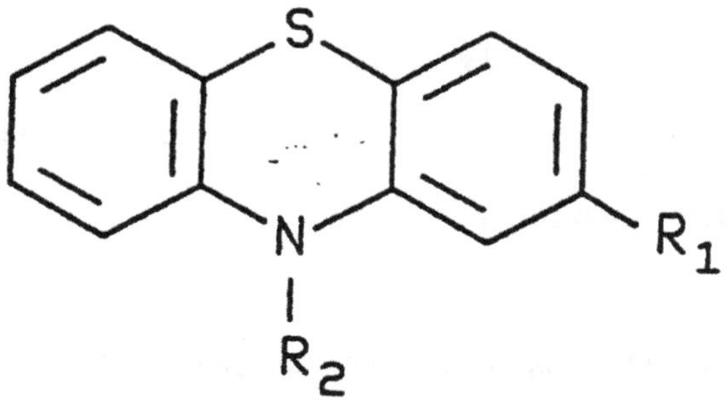

Figure 1: Tricyclic basic structure for phenothiazines

as can be seen in Figure 1. The important therapeutically useful phenothiazines are substituted in positions 2 and 10.

The 10' aminoalkyl phenothiazines are classified on the basis of their side chain: (5)

-Aliphatic substitution:

    (1) prototype activity: chlorpromazine.

    (2) pronounced sedative effects: most useful in agitated schizophrenics.

B-Piperidine group:

    (1) similar antipsychotic activity to chlorpromazine.

    (2) reduced extrapyramidal effects.

C-Piperazine group:

    (1) most potent antipsychotic activity.

    (2) insignificant sedative effects; therefore useful in depressed or withdrawn schizophrenics.

    (3) increased extrapyramidal effects.

Substitution at R1 includes:

A-Chlorine or methoxy group:

    (1) increased potency against psychotic behavior.

    (2) depression of motor activity.

B-Thiomethyl group:

    (1) increased potency against psychotic behavior.

C-Trifluoromethylene group:

    (1) greatly increased potency against psychotic behavior.

    (2) increased antiemetic potency.

    (3) increased tendency to produce extrapyramidal symptoms.

    (4) less sedation (6).

A summary of the structure-activity relationship is given in Table 1.

Pharmacology

The pharmacological properties of phenothiazines can be summarized as follows:

    1-sedation.

    2-decreased anxiety.

    3-decreased spontaneous motor activity.

    4-complex behavior is disrupted; difficulty with intellectual tasks.

    5-antihistaminic and hypotensive activity (1).

The above pharmacologic effects are thought to be mediated by the blockade of postsynaptic dopamine receptors resulting in an increase in the rate of production of dopamine metabolites and therefore interfering with the actions of dopamine as a synaptic neurotransmitter in the brain. (7)

Pharmacology and Clinical Applications of Acepromazine

Acepromazine (Promace, Atravet, Notensil) has most of the pharmacological effects typical of phenothiazines (8). It is generally considered more potent than chlorpromazine and promazine and is effective at very low doses. It has been shown that a dose of acepromazine as low as 0.1 mg/kg decreases the mean arterial blood pressure in dogs as well as in horses and in cats (9-13). The extent of hypotension seems to be dose independent since the same degree was observed with the high dose or low dose.

However, the duration of hypotension was much longer with the high dose (1.1 mg/kg) compared to a dose of 0.1 mg/kg (14).

In the dog, and to a lesser extent in the horse, acepromazine induces bradycardia due, most probably, to its adrenergic blocking actions (10). However, this bradycardia might be insignificant due to the reflex tachycardia induced by the hypotensive effects of the drug.

In the horse as well as the dog, acepromazine markedly decreases the respiratory rate (11, 15). This decrease in respiration rate, however, has no effect on either blood gases or blood pH. The most sensitive response to the action of acepromazine in the horse is the decrease in hematocrit or packed cell volume (PCV) (12). This effect is dose dependent and can be induced by a dose as small as 0.01 mg/kg . The decrease in hematocrit can be as high as 50 % and can last up to 12 hours with higher doses. The decrease in hematocrit is primarily due to a splenic sequestration of red blood cells.

Acepromazine is primarily used as a preanesthetic agent in the dog, cat and horse (15, 16, 18) . It markedly potentiates barbiturates facilitating handling and restraint of animals. Additionally, acepromazine is used in the treatment of equine colic (17). Partial blockade of adrenergic receptors may possibly explain this antispasmodic effect. Unfortunately, adequate blood volume and arterial pressure must exist before the drug can be administered because acepromazine can cause cardiovascular collapse or shock.

Acepromazine is not approved for use in cattle and should not be used in animals that are consumed by humans.

Toxicity of Acepromazine

The toxic reactions of phenothiazines can be divided into 3 types:

TABLE 1: Summary of the Structure-Activity Relationships of Phenothiazines

Drugs	Relative Potency	Sedative Effects	Antiemetic Effects	Adrenergic Antagonism	Extrapyramidal Effects[a]
Phenothiazines					
Dimethylaminopropyl	+[b]	+++	++	+++	Type I
Piperidine	+	++[c]	+	++	Infrequent
Piperazine	+++[d]	+	+++	+	Type I and II

a: Categories of extrapyramidal effects:

Type I: Motor restlessness or Parkinsonism or both after weeks or months of therapy.
Type II: Acute dystonic muscle spasms, particularly in young individuals early in treatment.

b: + means low or weak.

c: ++ means moderate.

d: +++ means high or strong.

A-Extrapyramidal effects:

    1-Parkinsonian syndrome: rigidity, tremors, etc...

    2-Akithisia: need for a constant motor activity.

    3-Dystonia: facial grimaces.

    4-Dyskinesia.

B-Sensitivity reactions:

    1-Jaundice.

    2-Dermatological reactions: rash, hives,
      photosensitivity.

C-Blood dyscriasias: leukocytosis (1).

In certain cases, sudden collapse has been observed manifested by apnea, slow pulse and unconsciousness. Some adverse behavioral alterations have been observed in the dog (19, 20). Aggression and vicious behavior have been manifested soon after administration (21). The CNS seizure threshold may be lowered leading to seizures in susceptible animals. Additionally, acepromazine can cause syncope associated with high vagal tone and subsequent bradycardia. In horses, acepromazine was noted to cause priapism or penile prolapse. This effect seems to be dose related and can last up to 10 hours with a dose of 0.4 mg/kg. The penile prolapse may be due in part to relaxation of the retractor penis muscles, which are innervated by adrenergic nerve fibers (22).

Metabolism

Both the phenothiazine nucleus and the side chain undergo substantial metabolic transformations (23-25). The main route of metabolism of the phenothiazines is by oxidation largely mediated by hepatic microsomal enzymes (26). Conjugation with glucuronic acid is very important. Most of these metabolites being very hydrophilic are excreted in the urine but to some extent also in the bile. Some of the phenothiazines have biologically active metabolites which complicate the correlation of concentrations in blood levels with biological effects (29). Scheme 1 summarizes the major metabolic pathways for the phenothiazine nucleus.

Concomitant with the metabolic changes in the nucleus, various biotransformations occur in the side chain, illustrated in Scheme 2. Sequentially, they are N-oxidation and hydroxylation, monodesmethylation, didesmethylation, desamination and beta-oxidation (28).

As for acepromazine specifically, the only reported study about its metabolism is by Dewey et al where they administered acepromazine to normal mares in the range of 5 to 50 mg. The major metabolite isolated from the urine of these horses was unconjugated 2(1-hydroxyethyl)promazine sulfoxide. Conjugated 7 hydroxy-acetylpromazine and conjugated 2-(1-hydroxyethyl)

7 hydroxy promazine were also isolated and identified. Additionally, 2(1-hydroxyethyl)promazine was isolated in some urine but in very minor quantities and thus the authors suggested that this route is very minor and can be considered negligible. Scheme 3 summarizes the metabolic scheme in the horse for acepromazine (30).

Pharmacokinetics

In general, pharmacokinetic studies of phenothiazines are few and usually inconclusive (31-37). In spite of the fact that the prototype, chlorpromazine, has been extensively studied; its renal excretion is almost totally unknown. To date, there is not a single report on the renal clearance of the parent drug or its metabolites in humans and animals.

The plasma concentration-time profiles usually follow a multiphasic pattern. Chlorpromazine has a large variation in the terminal half life (6.64 to 118.9 hours) in humans (31-37).

Large variations were also observed in the RBC/plasma concentration ratios (38, 39). Over 90 % of the phenothiazines in blood are bound to plasma proteins (40, 41).

There is only one pharmacokinetic study on acepromazine published to date (42). The drug was detectable up to 8 hours postinfusion after intravenous injection of a 0.3 mg/kg dose

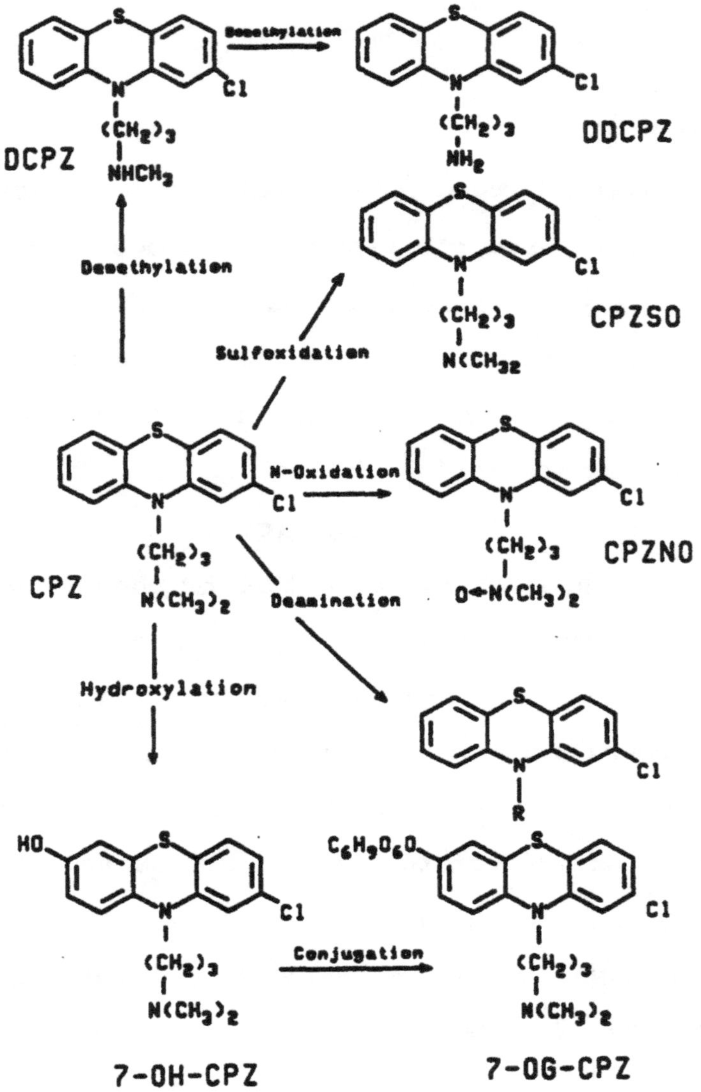

Principal metabolic reactions of chlorpromazine (CPZ).
DCPZ = demonomethylchlorpromazine; DDCPZ = dedimethyl-
chlorpromazine; 7-OH-CPZ = 7-hydroxychlorpromazine;
CPZSO = chlorpromazine sulphoxide; CPZNO = chlorpromazine N-
oxide; 7-OG-CPZ = 7-hydroxychlorpromazine glucuronide.
(Reprinted with permission, from Curry, 1976 b.)

Scheme I

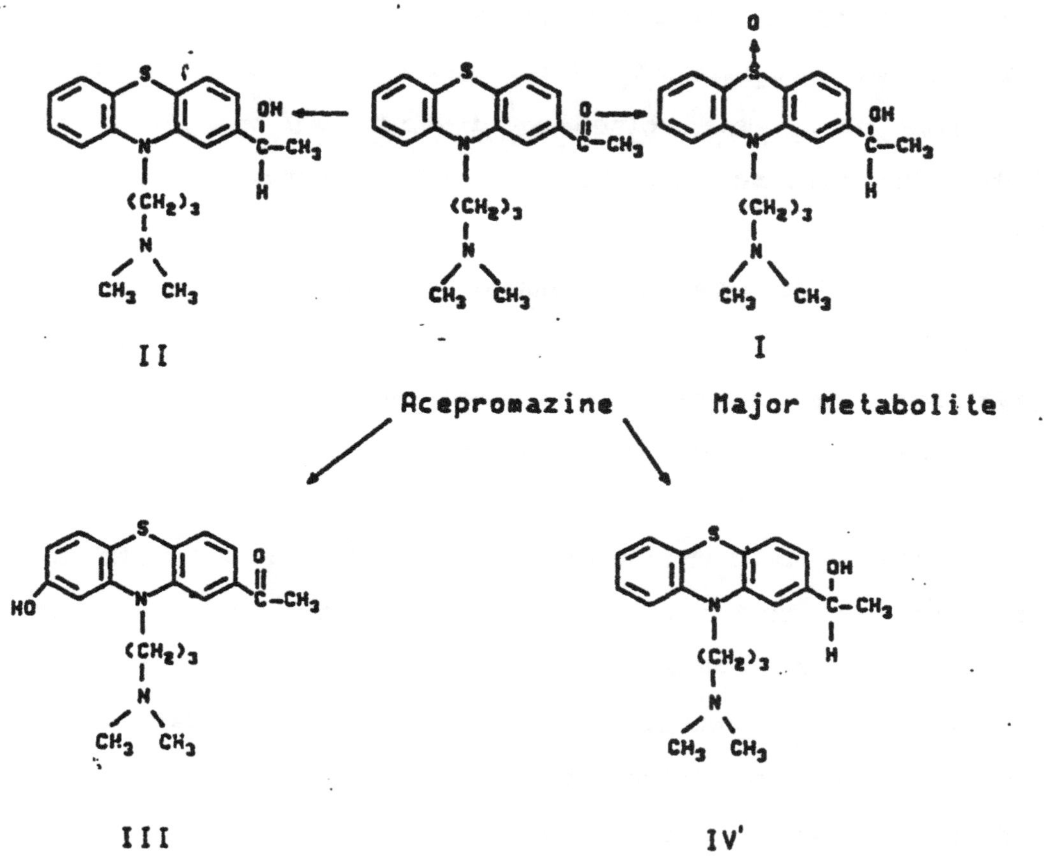

II

Acepromazine

I

Major Metabolite

III

IV'

III and IV were Isolated as Conjugates with Glucuronic Acid

Scheme II: Metabolic Pathways of Acepromazine in the Horse

of acepromazine. The plasma decay was biexponential with an alpha phase half life of 4.2 min and a beta phase half life of 184.8 min. The volume of distribution was 6.6 l/kg indicating that acepromazine was widely distributed in the horse.

It was also extensively bound to plasma proteins (> 99 %). In blood acepromazine partitioned in the plasma (46%) and in the erythrocyte phase (54%).

It is notable that, although that the study of Ballard and coworkers provided us with valuable information about the pharmacokinetics of this drug, the study's major drawback was the dose given to the horses. An acepromazine dose of 0.3 mg /kg is considered too high and will cause a lot of toxicities in the horse and therefore will be of little clinical value. Thus the need for other studies where a more clinically applicable dose is given and the results obtained would be of value to the practitioner in the clinic. The oral, subcutaneous and intramuscular bioavailability of acepromazine was not determined. For all these reasons, more thorough studies are needed to elucidate the pharmacokinetic properties of acepromazine.

Analytical Methods for the Assay of Phenothiazines

Successful pharmacokinetic studies depend on sensitive and specific analytical methods for both the parent compound and its metabolites.

Phenothiazines are difficult to assay because they are present in low quantities in body fluids. Their extreme lipophilicity leads to variable glass binding.

To date, various analytical methods have been described e.g. spectroscopy, fluorometry, radioimmunoassay, etc... (24) Sufficient specificity and appropriate sensitivity was achieved by Curry and Brodie in 1968 who assayed chlorpromazine at na

nogram levels (43-44) using a gas chromatograph equipped with an electron capture detector after extraction with heptane. Most of the subsequent published assays involved gas chromatography with either electron capture or nitrogen detectors with a lower limit of detection of 10 ng/ml. Although this limit has been satisfactory with the higher doses of phenothiazines, it was not enough for the more potent congeners.

There are 2 published assays for acepromazine to date, both using gas chromatography. Ballard and coworkers used GLC with a nitrogen detector. The column was 6 foot 3 % OV 101 glass column (42). The drug of interest was extracted from plasma with saturated tetrahydroborate buffer and dichloromethane (45).

Courtot used a flame ionization detection. The column was also 6 foot packed with either OV 1 or OV 17. Acepromazine was extracted from biological fluids mainly equine saliva with diethyl ether after alkalinization with 2 N NaOH. Unfortunately, in both these papers, no statistics were included and thus no conclusions about the sensitivities or the limit of detection could be drawn (46).

This dissertation presents a specific and sensitive assay for acepromazine using HPLC with an electrochemical detection.

CHAPTER 2

MATERIALS AND METHODS

Chemicals

Acetonitrile, hexane, ammonium acetate, sodium acetate, disodium phosphate and sodium hydrogen phosphate, sodium hydroxide, hydrochloric acid, toluene were LC or analytical grade from Fisher Scientific (Pittsburgh PA, USA). Hexamethyldisilazane- SCM Speciality Chemicals, Gainesville, Fla.

Acepromazine maleate as a powder was obtained from Fort Dodge Laboratories, Fort Dodge Iowa. Reference samples of marketed drugs were obtained from the manufacturers:

Chlorpromazine Hydrochloride, Trimeprazine Tartarate, Trifluoroperazine dihydrochloride- Smith Kline and French Laboratories, Philadelphia Pa.

Promethazine Hydrochloride- Aldrich Chemical Company, Milwauke Wisconsin.

Mesoridazine, Thioridazine Hcl- Sandoz Pharmaceuticals, E Hanover NJ.

Fluphenazine 2 Hcl- The Squibb Institute for Medical Research, Chicago Il.

Isoflurane-Forane, Anaquest, Madison, Wisconsin 53713

Na heparin-LyphoMed inc. Rosemont, Illinois 60018.

Polyflex (ampicillin suspension)- Avco Co., Inc., Fort Dodge, Iowa 50501.

0.9 % sodium chloride injection USP: Kendall McGaw Laboratories Inc. Irvine, Ca 92714.

Food

Purina Cat Chow: Ralston Purina Co., Saint Louis, Missouri 63164

General Apparatus:

Mettler Balance-Metler Instrument Corporation Hightstown N.J.

Metler Balance P1210-Metler Instrument Corporation Hightston N.J.

Tube Shaker-Eberbach Corporation, Ann Arbor Michigan.

Beckman Model TJ6 Centrifuge-Beckman Palo Alto Ca.

Microhematocrit Centrifuge-Damon/IEC Division, Needham Hts, Mass.

Microcapillary Reader-Damon/IEC Division, Needham Hts, Mass.

Micro-Hematocrit Capillary Tubes- Fisher Scientific, Pittsburgh Pa.

Thermolyne Maxi Mix 2 Mixer-Thermolyne Corporation, Dubuque Iowa.

Pierce Reacti-Therm Heating Module- Pierce Chemical Company, Rockford Illinois.

Corning pH Meter model 140- Corning Corporation Medfield, Mass.

CAry model 219 UV Spectrophotometer. Varian Corporation, Sugarland Texas.

Vacutainer- Vacutainer Systems, Rutherford, N.J.

Precision Microliter pipette Pipetman- Rainin Instrument Company, Woburn Mass.

Aquamatic K module K-20: American Medical Systems, Cincinnati Ohio 45238.

Vascular-Access-Port Model SLA with five French silicone rubber outlet catheter (0.8 mm ID and 1.7 mmOD):Access Technologies, Skokie, Illinois 60078.

Catheter Introducer:Becton Dickinson, Rutherford, New Jersey 07070.

Abbocath-T: Abbott Hospital inc, North Chicago, Illinois.

Angiocath 20 GA 2" #2818: Desert Medical Inc. Sandy Utah 84070.

Datascope Model 870: Datascope Corporation, Paramus, NJ 07653-0005.

P23-d model Transducer: Gold-Statham medical products division, Oxnard Ca 93030.

IL813 Blood gas and Acid-Base Analyzer: Instrumentation Laboratory Inc., Lexington Massachsetts.

The HPLC System consisted of:

-Waters Solvent Delivery System Model 6000- Waters Associates, Millford Mass.

-WISP automatic Injector Model 710 A- Waters Associates, Millford Mass.

-Data Module Model M730 - Waters Associates, Millford, Mass.

-Fisher Recordal 5000 series recorder- Fisher Scientific, Pittsburgh Pa.

-ESA Model 5100A Coulochem Electrochemical Detector-ESA Inc, Bedford, Mass.

The Oxidation Potential was set at .7 V for the Analytical Cell and .75 V for the Guard Cell.

The Column was a Zorbax Dupont CN bonded 13 cm column with a 5 um particle size diameter Obtained from Mac-Mod Analytical Inc, Chadds Ford, Pa.

The mobile phase consisted of either 90:10 acetonitrile: .2 M ammonium acetate pH 6.9 or 75:25 acetonitrile: 0.1 M acetate buffer pH 4.75. The only exception for these conditions was with mesoridazine where the mobile phase consisted of 75:25 acetonitrile 0.1 M phosphate buffer pH 6.

The flow rate was 1.2 ml/min.

Stability Studies of Acepromazine in Water and 1 N HCl

Five mls of a 0.1 mg/ml aquous stock solution of acepromazine were added to two tubes, one containing 45 mls of pure deionized water, the other, 1 N HCl so that the final concentration was 10 ug/ml. These solutions were covered by aluminum foil to protect them from the ultraviolet light and were incubated at 90 ° C. The UV absorbance of various aliquots of these cooled (t0 room temperature) incubated solutions taken at different times were measured.

The spectrophotometric settings were:

-scan rate: 2 nm/sec.

-chart speed: 10 nm/sec.

-range: 500-200 nm.

-the full scale of the recorder was 1 absorbance unit.

Determination of the Partition coefficient between Hexane and Phosphate Buffer pH 7.4 for Some Selected Phenothiazines

Seven solutions of the different phenothiazines (thioridazine, fluphenazine, chlorpromazine, trifluoroperazine, mesoridazine, acepromazine, promazine) were prepared by adding 0.1 ml of a 100 ug/ml aquous stock solution to 10 mls of phosphate buffer pH 7.4. The concentration of each solution was measured by HPLC before and after extraction with various volumes of hexane ranging from 0.1 ml to 10 mls (0.1 ml for thioridazine, chlorpromazine, trifluoroperazine, promazine, 1 ml for acepromazine and fluphenazine and 10 mls for mesoridazine).

Additionally, 0.5 ml of the hexane were taken and dried under a constant stream of nitrogen and reconstituted in mobile phase.

The concentration of the phenothiazine in the buffer andthe mobile phase was determined by HPLC from a standard calibration curve in buffer and mobile phase respectively.

The partition coefficient was determined in 2 ways:

$$D = [C_h]/[C_{bu}] \qquad (1)$$

where C_h is the concentration in hexane and C_{bu} is the concentration in buffer solution, and

$$D = (([C_b]_b - [C_b]_e)/([C_b]_e)) \times (V_e/V_o) \qquad (2)$$

where $[C_b]_b$ is the buffer concentration before extraction, $[C_b]_e$ is the buffer concentration after extraction, V_e is the volume of the aqueous phase, and V_o is the volume of the organic phase.

Analysis of Acepromazine and Other Phenothiazines from Biological Fluids Mainly Plasma, Urine and Whole Blood

To a sample of 0.5 to 2ml of biological fluid such as plasma, urine or whole blood 0.1 mls of 1 N NaOH are added to make the pH alkaline. An appropriate amount of a suitable sample is added. This alkaline sample is then extracted with 5 mls of hexane for 1 hour. After centrifugation, the hexane phase was removed and evaporated to dryness at 25°C under a constant stream of nitrogen. If any emulsion still persisted after centrifugation, gentle stirring with a glass rod followed by further centrifugation solved the problem. The residue was redissolved in an appropriate volume of mobile phase usually 250 ul and an aliquot of this reconstituted residue was injected into the chromatographic system.

Red Blood Cell/Plasma Distribution Coefficient

Since phenothiazines as a class have a relatively high lipophilicity, it seems that a distribution between red blood cells (rbc) and plasma would occur when the drugs were introduced into a volume of whole blood. To analyze for such disribution, the red blood cell concentration/plasma ratio was determined.

From fresh blood obtained from the blood bank, packed rbcs was obtained by centrifugation, these rbcs was washed three times with isotonic saline and finally resuspended in isotonic phosphate buffer pH 7.4.

Either these pseudoblood samples or whole blood was spiked with different amounts of the phenothiazine of interest so that the final concentration is 300, 500 and 1000 ng/ml respectively. The hematocrit was measured after equilibration of the samples for 60 minutes at 37°C.

After centrifugation for 20 minutes at 3000 rpm, the hematocrit of the red blood cell phase was measured to determine how much supernatant was left after centrifugation. Additionally, an aliquot of the rbc phase was taken and diluted with equal amounts of water in order to lyse the cells so that it was possible to measure their drug content.

Both the supernatant phase and the rbc phase were analyzed for their drug content.

Appropiate calibration curves in both supernatant and rbc were constructed by spiking blank supernatant and blank rbc solutions with different amounts of the corresponding phenothiazine and the internal standard so that the final concentrations would be between 1000 ng/ml and 25 ng/ml.

RBC partitioning was evaluated in 3 different ways:

$$D = [C_{rbc}]/[C_{pw}] \quad (3)$$

$$C_{rbc}/C_{pw} = [(A_{tot} - (C_{pw} * V_{pw}))/(V_b * H]/C_{pw} \quad (47) \quad (4)$$

$$D = (C_{rbc} - (Cp_w(1-H))/(H/Cp_w) \quad (5)$$

where D is the RBC-supernatant partitioning coefficient, C_{rbc} is the concentration of the drug in the red blood cells, C_{pw} is the concentration of the drug in the supernatant, A_{tot} is the total amount of drug added to the blood or pseudoblood, Vb is the volume of blood or pseudoblood, Vpw is the volume of supernatant calculated as (1-Hb)*Vb with Hb being the hematocrit of the blood

or pseudoblood before spiking with the drug solution and H is the hematocrit of the red blood cell phase after separation of the two phases.

Concentration dependency of the red blood cell partitioning for the various phenothiazines was challenged by determining this coefficient at various concentrations mainly at 1000, 500 and 300 ng/ml respectively.

The three results calculated from the three different methods were compared to determine significant glass binding and the extent it affected the results.

Extent of Protein Binding Calculated from the Red Blood Cell Partitioning Studies

The extent of protein binding was calculated from the differences between the red blood cell partition coefficients between plasma and the red blood cells and between phosphate buffer and red blood cells. The fraction of drug bound to proteins was calculated from:

$$f = 1 - Kd/D \quad (47)$$

where f is the fraction of drug bound to proteins, Kd is the red blood cells partition coefficient between plasma and the red blood cell phase, D is the red blood cell partition coefficient between the phosphate buffer and the red blood cells. This extent of protein binding was determined at a concentration of 1 ug/ml.

Bioavailabilty of Acepromazine in the Cat

Experimental Animals

The studies performed were approved in advance by the University of Florida's Institutional Animal Use and Care Committee. The laboratory facilities were also approved by that committee for the performance of minor survival surgical procedures including placement of the vascular access ports.

The animals used in these studies were adult male short haired domestic cats with an average age of 12.6 +/- 0.44 months (range: 6-33) and which weighed an average 4.2 +/- 0.55 Kg (range:2.6-5.8). The cats were purchased from a USDA Licensed Animal Dealer who had bred the cats in a minimal disease colony.

Following the investigators' stipulations, none of the cats had received any drugs or medical treatment other than routine vaccinations as kittens and, in the housing at the University of Florida.

The cats were housed and maintained in the University of Florida's Health Center Animal Resources Division's facilities which are approved by the American Association for the Accreditation of Laboratory Animal Care. The cats were fed commercial dry cat food ad libitum and water.

Vascular Access Port Implantation

Frequent blood sampling required direct access to the systemic venous system. This was acheived by implanting vascular ports into the femoral and jugular vein of the cat which allowed percutaneous access.

Norfolk Vascular Access Port:

The unit implanted consisted of a silicone rubber cathether connected to a blind reservoir. The reservoir was encased at its base and sides in a more rigid plastic which had flanges and holes to facilitating in anchoring it in the body. The top of the reservoir was a rubber septum through which access can be got to the bore of the catheter. The catheter itself can be of varied sizes but a 5 French gauge (1.7 mm OD and 0.8 mm ID) catheter was chosen for insertion into the cat's femoral vein. The catheter was shipped by the manufacturer at a 12 cm length. The size port used for insertion in the cat was the SLA model with a reservoir approximately 15 mm in diameter and 10 mm in height.

Upon receipt of the catheter from the manufacturer it was wiped with alcohol and washed with soapy water to remove any grease or foreign material. It was then tested by injecting distilled water through the reservoir and occluding the distal end of the catheter whilst pressurizing the system. Leaks would then be visible. No leaks were seen in new ports but were found in occasional ports that had been removed from animals and were being recycled. Approximately 15 to 17 cm from the reservoir, a bead of silicone rubber sealant was placed around the catheter to allow suturing of the catheter to the vessel it was being implanted into without risking damage to the catheter itself. The bead was allowed to cure for 24 hours. The ports were then thoroughly washed with distilled water and packaged for autoclaving.

Implantation of the Port

The cats were anesthesized (usually with isoflurane). Once anesthetized, and at a surgical plane of anesthesia, the medial and lateral left thigh was prepared for aseptic surgery. The port to be implanted was flushed with heparinized saline (1 IU heparin /ml 0.9 % saline for injection USP).

With the cat in right lateral recumbency, the left leg was raised and a stab incision made through the skin just medial to the patella. A pair of long hemostats was then passed through the incision, tunneling subcutaneously upwards to the lateral flank where a skin incision was made to exteriorize the tips.

The distal end of the vascular access port's catheter was grasped by the hemostats and the catheter drawn subcutaneously to emerge at the knee incision. Sufficient catheter was drawn through the subcutaneous tunnel so that the reservoir was pulled against the skin. The cat was rolled into lateral recumbency of the opposite side exposing the sterile prepared groin area.

The femoral vein was palpated high in the cat's groin and a 2-4 cm incision made over it. The fascia covering the femoral vein , nerve and artery lifted away and dissected. The femoral vein was separated from the accompanying femoral nerve and artery. Two pieces of suture were looped under the vein to facilitate lifting it and ocluding it during puncture and initial catheter insertion. At this time a subcutaneous tunnel was made down to the knee incision to bring the the catheter up to the exposed vein. The silicone rubber catheter was then cut so it was 5 cm long from bead to tip. The cut was done with a scalpel blade so the catheter had an untraumatized bevel of about 45. It was important that the tip not be roughened or damaged as it was thought that such a damage could act as a nidus for a thrombus formation.

When all preparations were complete, the vein was raised and the proximal suture used to occlude the vein. A 19 gauge needle was then placed at an acute angle cranially into the vein to the extent that about half the bevel had entered the vein and then it was withdrawn. To confirm penetration into the venous lumen, the proximal suture loop was momentarily lowered so blood could flow from the puncture site. A venous dilator was then placed into the puncture hole and moved up in the venous lumen. The catheter was grasped lightly with blunt forceps and passed under the dilator into the vein towards the heart. As the catheter approached the proximal suture, the loop was relaxed whereupon usually some visible confirmation of placement could be seen as a faint blood pulse wave in the catheter lumen. The catheter was then rapidly passed up the remainder of its length until the bead reached the venous puncture site. The bleb was sutured to the artery wall and surrounding fascial and muscle tissue. The groin wound was closed.

The cat was returned to lateral recumbency and the reservoir sutured to muscle fascia under a skin pocket and the skin wound closed. The cat was given ampicillin antibiotic coverage prophylactically for the next three days.

Maintenance of the Vascular Port

The vascular access port was maintained by a heparin lock that was removed and replaced, two to three times a week, after first flushing vigorously with physiological saline. All injections into or out of the port were performed aseptically.

Administration, Collection and Treatment of Samples:

The bioavailabilty of Acepromazine in the cat after oral, intramuscular and subcutaneous as compared to intravenous administration was studied as following:
The study was a cross over design whereby each animal served as his own control.

Initially, two cats were given 0.3 mg/kg of acepromazine IV (the concentration of the solution was 0.5 mg/ml). The two other cats were each given orally a 10 mg tablet. After a washout period of two weeks the treatments were switched so that the first two cats received the oral treatment and the second two cats received the IV treatment. After a period of approximately three weeks, the same four cats were administered a dose of 0.3 mg/kg subcutaneously and 0.3 mg/kg IM with a washout period of three to four weeks in between treatments.

Two mls of blood were withdrawn from the implanted port per sampling time. The hematocrit for each blood sample was measured. After the hematocrit measurement, the blood sample was centrifuged immediately at 300 rpm to separate plasma and red blood cells.

After each blood sample withdrawal, the cats were reinjected with 2 mls of isotonic saline solution to prevent hypovolemia and shock in the cats.

The initial protocol for blood sampling after IV administration was: 0, 1.5, 3, 4.5, 6, 7.5, 9, 12, 15, 18, 24, 30, 45, 60, 75, 90, 120, 150, 180, 210, 240, 300, and 360 minutes respectively.

The protocol for PO, SQ and IM was modified so that the sampling times were as following: 0, 4, 8, 12, 16, 20, 23, 26, 30, 35, 40, 50, 60, 75, 90, 120, 150, 180, 210, 240, 300, 360 minutes respectively.

No urine was collected from these cats since catheterization of unsedated cats was not possible.

Prior to experimentation, the animals were given enough time to acclimate to their surroundings. Their full medical history was well characterised.

Pharmacodynamics-Pharmacokinetics of Acepromazine in the Horse

All these studies were conducted using seven donated horses whose medical histories are summarized in Appendix 1.

These horses were given each 0.15 mg/kg of acepromazine intravenously (the concentration of the solution was 0.5 mg/ml).

The acepromazine was injected into the right jugular vein through an 18 gauge two inch teflon over-the-needle catheter. Blood samples for acepromazine assay were withdrawn from the left jugular vein through a 14 G five inch teflon over the-needle catheter. Both catheters were kept flushed with heparinized saline. The sampling protocol was exactly the same one used in the iv cat studies. The hematocrit and the blood samples were treated the same way as described in the cat studies.

The following pharmacodynamics parameters were measured as described in the following:

Blood Pressure Measurements

Systemic systolic, diastolic and mean blood pressures were obtained by transducing the pressures obtained by the percutaneous cathaterization of the transfacial artery. The artery was cannulated with a 20 G two inch over-the-needle catheter and this was connected to a pressure transducer by means of a physiological saline filled pressure manometer tube. The transducer was powered by a multichannel oscilloscope with digital pressure and heart rate displays. After an adequate warm-up period was allowed to elapse, the transducer system was calibrated against a mercury column manometer at zero (atmospheric pressure only), 50, 100, 150 and 200 mm Hg.

Heart Rate

Heart rate was determined by the rate counter on the multichannel oscilloscope that counted the number of arterial pulse wave per ten second period and gave a beats per minute count output.

Blood Gas ANalysis

Systemic arterial blood gas tensions and pH were measured from samples collected anaerobically from the arterial catheter into a heparinized plastic syringe. The sample was placed into either an IL813 or IL1304 Blood Gas Analyzer within two hours minutes of collection. Immediately after collection the sample was stoppered and stored in ice slush until analysis could be performed.

The blood gas analyzer was calibrated each according to the manufacturer's instructions with two sets of standards.

Additionally the analyzer's performance was checked on the day of each study with the manufacturer's quality control samples.

Electrocardiogram

Electrocardiographic (ECG) tracings were obtained using Lead II where the left and right arm electrodes were placed laterally at the level of the shoulder and about three inches caudal to it on the left and right sides respectively, while the leg electrode was placed on the left thorax at the level of the 10th rib about 5 inches lateral to the spinal column. The "electrodes" were commercial pre-jelled self-sticking electrodes placed on skin that had been thoroughly cleaned with isopropyl alcohol. The ECG was displayed on the multichannel analyzer described above.

Urinary Catheter

The mare's urinary bladders were cathetherized using sterile 30 G French Foley catheters placed by manual palpation. The catheters balloons were inflated using water and a weight tied to the catheter to keep it lodged against the neck of the bladder. The catheters were attached to plastic collection bags which were emptied into measuring cylinders when required so urine output was to be measured. The urine tended not to be free flowing and was usually obtained by stimulating the mare to urinate by manipulating the catheter.

Venous Sampling Line

The hair is clipped over the jugular groove mid neck and the skin sterilized with alcohol.

A 14 gauge 5.25 inch catheter was placed in the jugular vein. On the other side of the neck the same procedure was repeated but with 18 gauge 2 inch catheter. An adhesive ECG electrode was placed and patched over each shoulder and on the mid left thorax. These electrodes were connected using an ECG lead II configuration. A strain-gauge pressure transducer was connected to the oscilloscope and allowed to warm up 20 minutes then calibrated against a mercury column manometer. A 20 gauge 2 inch catheter was placed in either the transfacial or ocular artery and connected through a saline filled manometer tubing to a strain gauge transducer.

CNS and Sedative Effects

The sedative and central nervous system effects were evaluated by rating the degree of sedation, the general behavior, the posture and the general alertness of the horse according to a scale developped jointly by the principal investigators. This scale or rating is presented in appendix 2.

All the horses were rated by the same person to avoid any subjective differences from one person to the other.

Evaluation and Fitting of Pharmacokinetic Data

The observed plasma concentrations of acepromazine were separately fitted using a commercial softwear package (RSTRIP) to a sum of exponentials and also using the Lotus 123 spreadsheet.

In the case of first order input and excretion, the linear sum of exponentials were fitted to:

$$C = A_1 e^{-k_1 t} + A_2 e^{-k_2 t}$$

where C is the expected value of plasma concentration, Ai and Ki are constants and t is time in minutes. Methods for estimating Ai and Ki were discussed by Riggs (47) and Gibaldi and Perrier (48). The methods of analysis of weighted residual and weighted residual sum of squares were used to minimize the number of exponentials and obtain the best estimates of each Ai and Ki. The residuals could be defined as the difference between estimated values of C and the observed values at a given time.

The absorption rate constants were determined using the Loo-Riegelman method (49) where the fraction absorbed or the fraction remaining to be absorbed is plotted vs time.

The bioavailabity of acepromazine was determined by comparing the areas under the plasma concentration time curve for the different routes of administration with the area after intravenous administration after adjusting for the different doses.

Pharmacokinetic Symbols and Definitions

Alpha: distribution rate constant (min^{-1}) describing the distribution of the drug from the central compartment to peipheral tissues in the body.

Beta: disposition rate constant (min^{-1}) summarizing the complexity of elimination and re-equilibration that describes the ultimate disposition of the drug in the central compartment.

C0: plasma concentration at time 0 (ng/ml).

MRT: mean residence time (minutes). It represents the time for 63.2% of the administered dose to be eliminated

Vdss: volume of distribution at steady state (liters). This volume relates drug concentration in plasma or blood to the total amount of drug in the body during steady state.

Vdpss: volume of distribution at pseudo steady state (liters). It is an estimate of the volume of distribution on the assumption of a one compartment body model when in fact you have two compartments and is usually an overestimate of the volume of distribution. This volume relates drug concentration in plasma or blood to the total amount of drug in the body during the terminal exponential phase for any multicompartment model where elimination occurs from the central compartment.

Vdcc: volume of distribution of central compartment (liters). This volume term may be useful for estimating peak concentrations in plasma or blood for drugs that distribute relatively slowly in the body and are absorbed relatively rapidly after oral or intramuscular administration.

Cltot: clearance total (ml/min). It is the hypothetical volume of blood that is completly cleared from the drug per unit of time.

Calculation of the Various Pharmacokinetic Parameters

$MRT = AUMC_{00}/AUC_{00}$

$Vdcc = Dose/C0$

$Vdpss = Cltot/beta$

$Vdss = Cltot*MRT$

$Cltot = Dose/AUC_{00}$

$AUC_{trap}(tn) = \text{sum } i=1 \text{ to } n \ ((c_i + c_{i-1})*(t_i - t_{i-1})/2)$

$AUMC_{trap}(tn) = \text{sum} i=1 \text{ to} n((c_i*t_i + c_{i-1}*t_{i-1})*(t_i - t_{i-1})/2)$

$AUC_{extra} = c_n/beta.$

$$AUMC_{extra} = c_n * t_n/beta + c_n/beta^2$$

$$AUC_{00} = AUC_{trap}(t_n) + AUC_{extra}$$

$$AUMC_{00} = AUMC_{trap}(t_n) + AUMC_{extra}$$

CHAPTER 3

RESULTS AND DISCUSSION

Analysis of Acepromazine in Plasma, Whole Blood and Red Blood Cells

The HPLC chromatogram of blank plasma and plasma containing 100 ng/ml acepromazine with trimeprazine (150 ng/ml) from a cat receiving 0.3 mg /kg of acepromazine IV is shown in Figure 2 . At worst the coefficient of variation on repeated assay of plasma containing known quantities of acepromazine was 16.5 % . At best this value was 3.89 %. The type of calibration curve presented in Figure 3 is

$$y= -0.01044+/-0.0279 + (0.595+/-0.0258)x$$

where y is the peak height ratio and x is the concentration of acepromazine in the plasma. The correlation coefficient was 0.9943. The reproducibilty of analysis for interday and intraday variability is shown in tables 2 and 3 respectively. The acpromazine was reproducibly recovered (see Table 4).

The coefficient of variation is relatively high. This is due to the fact that phenothiazines being very lipophilic exhibit a large degree of glass binding and this renders their assay more difficult due to the introduction of a large degree of variabilty from assay to assay.

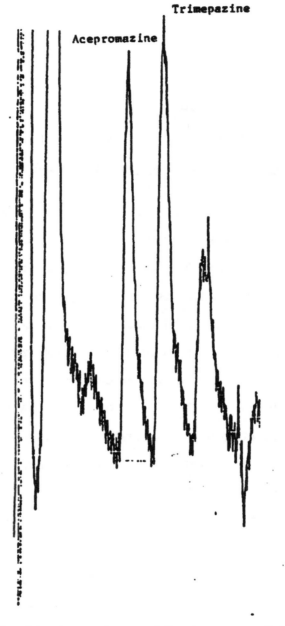

Figure 2: Liquid chromatographic traces of blank cat plasma and cat plasma containing 100 ng/mL of Acepromazine with trimepazine (150 ng/mL)

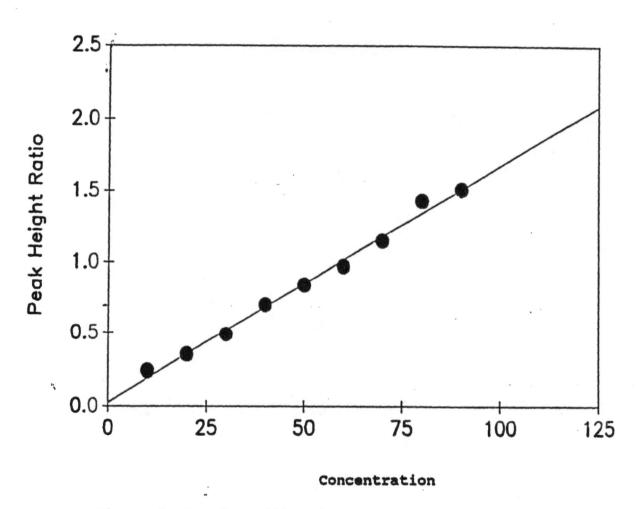

Figure 3 Sample calibration curve for the HPLC assay of Acepromazine

Table 2: Interday Variability For The HPLC Assay of Acepromazine Maleate
From Biological Fluids

AMONG DAYS VARIABILITY

CONC	PEAK HEIGHT RATIO					
(ng/ml)	R1	R2	R3	MEAN	SD	CV(%)
100	1.57	1.69	1.59	1.61	0.06	3.99
90	1.33	1.41	1.41	1.38	0.05	3.33
80	-	1.17	1.26	-	-	-
70	1.06	1.05	1.11	1.07	0.03	3.00
60	0.83	0.93	0.96	0.91	0.07	7.50
50	0.71	0.87	0.80	0.79	0.08	10.3
40	0.65	0.72	0.65	0.67	0.04	5.94
30	0.33	0.55	0.50	0.46	0.11	25.07
20	0.29	0.35	0.35	0.33	0.03	10.44
10	0.21	0.27	0.20	0.22	0.04	17.20

Table 3: Intraday Variability For The HPLC Assay of Acepromazine Maleate From Biological Fluids.

WITHIN DAY VARIABILITY

CONC (ng/mL)	PEAK HEIGHT RATIO						
	R1	R2	R3	R4	MEAN	SD	CV(%)
100	1.32	1.43	1.59	2.17	1.44	0.13	9.42
90	1.54	1.43	1.41	1.51	1.47	0.06	4.24
80	1.31	1.24	1.26	1.43	1.31	0.08	6.50
70	1.18	1.08	1.11	1.15	1.13	0.04	3.89
60	1.10	0.97	0.96	0.97	1.00	0.06	6.60
50	0.83	0.77	0.80	0.84	0.81	0.03	3.90
40	0.74	0.70	0.65	0.69	0.69	0.04	5.30
30	0.47	0.34	0.50	0.49	0.45	0.07	16.5
20	0.40	0.30	0.35	0.35	0.35	0.04	11.6
10	0.22	0.20	0.20	0.24	0.21	0.02	8.90

Table 4: The Extraction Recovery of Acepromazine From Biological Fluids

CONC (ng/ml)	R1[a]	R2	R3	R4	MEAN	SD[b]	CV(%)[c]
100	82	93.04	101.04	113.45	97.38	11.47	11.78
90	96.5	93.1	90.42	80.84	90.21	5.82	6.45
80	81.14	80.47	80.58	76.95	79.78	1.65	2.07
70	72.7	70.04	71.26	63.15	69.29	3.66	5.29
60	67.35	63.3	56.9	54.44	60.5	5.1	8.44
50	49.6	50.21	50.87	47.79	49.62	1.14	2.31
40	43.7	45.41	33.07	40.74	40.73	4.72	11.6
30	26.04	21.83	27.19	30.74	26.45	3.18	12.02
20	21.69	19.37	20.71	23.65	21.35	1.56	7.3
10	9.29	13.21	17.93	18.23	14.66	3.68	25.15

[a]Refers to replicate assays. [b]Standard deviation. [c]Coefficient of variation.

TABLE 5: Summary of the Equations Describing the Calibration Curve for Each Phenothiazine Assayed by the HPLC System.

DRUG	SLOPE	SESa	INTERCEPT	SEIb	R
ACEPROMAZINE	0.72	0.03	0.133	0.046	0.993
PROCHLOPERAZINE	1.85	0.16	−0.07	0.05	0.988
FLUPHENAZINE	0.007	0.0005	0.686	0.68	0.992
THIORIDAZINE	0.0036	0.0002	0.408	0.135	0.989
TRIFLUOROPERAZINE	0.0002	0.0001	0.017	0.005	0.993
MESORIDAZINE	0.18	0.009	0.033	0.047	0.994
PROMAZINE	0.002	0.00013	0.07	0.12	0.984
CHLORPROMAZINE	8.41	0.194	−0.155	0.178	0.997

Analysis of Other Phenothiazines in Plasma, Whole Blood and Red Blood Cells

In general all the 6 other phenothiazines studied for their red blood cell partitioning were analyzed using the same chromatographic conditions as described for acepromazine. Their retention times ranged between 6 and 12 minutes respectively. The equations of the calibration curve for each drug are summarized in Table 5. The extraction procedures with hexane were exactly as described for acepromazine except for mesoridazine which is more polar and had to be extracted with toluene.

Stability of Acepromazine in 1 N NaOH and 1 N HCl at 90 ^{0} C

Acepromazine was found to be stable from acid and base degradation for up to 24 hours at 90 ^{0} centigrade since there was no significant change in its concentration as measured by UV. Thus, for our purposes acepromazine can be considered stable enough for analysis.

Partition Coefficient Between Hexane and Phosphate Buffer pH 7.4 for some Clinically Relevant Phenothiazines

The apparent partition coefficients between hexane and phosphate buffer pH 7.4 were determined by measuring the concentration in the aqueous and organic phase and by differences in the concentrations in the aqueous phase before and after extraction. The results are summarized in Table 6. As expected mesoridazine, being a polar metabolite of thioridazine had the lowest partitioning in hexane (K=.0141). The most lipophilic was trifluoroperazine (K= 193) which had a partitioning slightly higher than thioridazine or chlorpromazine (K=129-152). Fluphenazine and acepromazine could be considered of intermediate lipophilicity with a partition coefficient of around 10.

It is to be noted that greater variability in the results was observed with the more lipophilic phenothiazines, ie thioridazine and chlorpromazine. This is most probably due to the fact that the more lipophilic the phenothiazine, the greater is the glass binding thus introducing more difficulty and more variabilty into assessment techniques.

Lipophilicity and Red Blood Cell Partitioning

It is an established fact that lipid solubility is a very important factor in the actions of drugs affecting the brain and central nervous system. Thus for a drug to exert its pharmacological activity in the brain it should be able to cross the blood brain barrier. Fundamentally, the more lipid soluble the drug is, the more likely and the easier it is to cross this barrier (50).

This is the basis of the Ferguson principle concerning central nervous depressants which states that the depressant effect of unrelated substances increases with increasing oil-water partition coefficient. In other words, the higher the partition coefficient, the greater the depressant action. However, this relationship is not linear but parabolic because substances that are very lipophilic will accumulate first in oily sites of loss and will be trapped there and will not be able to exert their action in the targetted tissues.

This is typically exemplified by the barbiturates. Thiopental, the most lipophilic of the group enters the brain most rapidly after IV injection. An intermediate rate of penetration is shown by amobarbital. Relatively polar barbiturates such as barbital penetrate the brain quite slowly such that it has no utility in clinical situations.

The influence of lipid solubility is not limited to brain penetration. It is a factor in absorption from the gastrointestinal tract, reabsorption in the renal tubule and in metabolism. Metabolism itself confers polarity but there is a stong evidence that a certain level of lipophilicity is needed if a drug is to bind to microsomal P-450 enzymes. This fact raises the question of whether other binding reactions are similarly related. Indeed, binding to plasma proteins often correlates with lipophilicity as if the chemistry controlling lipophilicity also controls binding affinity. For instance, there is a nearly perfect correlation between the binding of some phenothiazines to bovine serum albumin and the octanol/pH 7.4 buffer logarithm of the partition coefficient (51). Binding to dopamine receptors of the D-2 type also correlates with lipid solubilty and therefore with protein binding. However, 7 hydroxychlorpromazine has pharmacological activity in excess of that predicted from its lipid solubility. In contrast, the plasma protein binding of this active metabolite is considerably below that of the parent compound and below the inactive chlorpromazine N oxide. Presumably, the hydroxyl group inhibits the entry of the molecule into the hydrophobic interior of the albumin molecule. Therefore lipid solubility and protein binding seem to be poor predictors of potency. It was thought that the ease or ability of a drug to enter or partition into the RBCs would correlate well with the ability of the drug to cross the blood brain barrier and enter the brain. Thus the RBC partition coefficient might be a better indicator or predictor of the potency of phenothiazines. For that purpose the relationship between red blood cell partitioning and lipophilicity was investigated. The red blood cell partition

coefficients for the various phenothiazines studied as a
function of concentration are summarized in Table 7. Figure
4 shows the plot of the red blood cell partition as a function
of lipophilicity for the phenothiazines of interest at the
three concentartions investigated.

As can be seen this partition coefficient for all the
phenothiazines studied except for mesoridazine lie within the
same values. Typically, the red blood partition coefficient
was around five which meant that these phenothiazines were
mostly found in the red blood cells. It was also observed
that these values were independent of the concentration (see
analysis of variance in Table 8). These results are contrary
to what was expected because it was thought that that the more
lipophilic the phenothiazine is the easier it is going to bind
or partition into the red blood cell. The nondependence of
this partitioning on lipophilicity might be explained by the
fact that at pH 7.4 all these phenothiazines having a pKa of
9 (being basic amines) will be in the ionized form. The
existence of the positive charge on the amine will impart a
certain degree of polarity which will be the same for this
class of drugs and thus it will overule the lipophilicity
parameter in partitioning. Thus because of the positive
charge they will most probably have the same physical

characteristics and thus will all partition in the same way.
Another reason for the nondependence of the red blood cell
partitioning on lipophilicity might be due to the fact that
the drug is not partitioning into the cell itself but binding
to either the membrane or to some component inside the cell.
In this case, lipophilicity will not be a major factor in
contributing to the magnitude of this partition coefficient
and other factors will play a much more important role since
hydrophylic compounds can also be bound to the membrane of
the cell and thus will have a relatively large red blood cell
partition coefficient (greater than 1). It is noteworthy to
mention that Ballard and coworkers found out that the red
blood cell coefficient was around 11. This value was
calculated from the protein binding which was found to be 90
% at a concentration of 1000 ng/ml and the partition
coefficient in whole blood at the same concentration which was
found to be 1.12. The value that Ballard obtained seem to be
excessively large since it was almost double than what we had
obtained in our studies.

It is notable that for drugs that are very lipophilic and
that exhibit a great degree of glass binding, the red blood
cell partition coefficient cannot be calculated by just
measuring the concentration in the buffer phase and

calculating the concentration or amount in the red blood cells by difference. This will result in an overestimation of the red blood cell coefficient as it is seen and confirmed from the results obtained in our studies. This overestimation is due to the fact that the drug that is not found in the supernatant phase is assumed to be bound to the red cells. However, for drugs that undergo glass binding, there is a three way partition between the glass, the red blood cells and the glass walls. From the results presented in Table 7, it can be seen that the red blood cell partition coefficient was overestimated for the phenothiazines studied as compared to the value obtained by the actual mesurement of both phases. This overestimation was almost 100 % in certain cases such as thioridazine where the partition coefficient was 6.3 by actual measurement and 11.8 by difference.

On the other hand, the red blood cell partition coefficient can be underestimated if it is assumed that the red blood cell phase is completely made of red blood cells and there was no plasma water present between the cells. It was found that the red blood cells phase is not made of 100 % red cells but that around 10 to 20 % of the volume was plasma water. This resulted in an underestimation of the concentration in the red blood cell phase because the concentration measured was a combination of the concentration in the blood cells and the concentration in the plasma water. This underestimation is found only in the case where the drugs partition highly in the red blood cells such as seen with the phenothiazines because the actual concentration measured is smaller than what the concentration would be if the red blood cell phase was completely or 100 % red cells.

On the other hand, an overestimation would result for drugs that would poorly partition in the red blood cells because the concentration measured would be higher than the actual value if it is assumed that the red blood cell phase is only red cells because more drug would be present per unit volume in the plasma phase than the red cell phase.

Extent of Protein Binding

The extent of protein binding for the phenothiazines studied are summarized in Table 9. The fraction bound was determined at a concentration of 1000 ng/ml. The results obtained agree with what was reported in the litterature for at least one compound promazine using totally different methods.

As for the other phenothiazines, no information was available for their protein binding was available at the concentration range studied. From our studies acepromazine

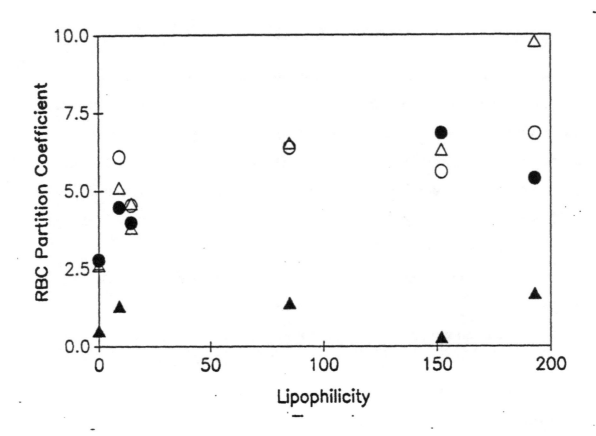

Figure 4: Plot of the red blood cell partition coefficient vs lipophilicity for the phenothiazine of interest. (◯) 300 ng/ml; (●) 500 ng/ml; (△) 1000 ng/ml; (▲) whole blood 1000 ng/ml.

Table 6: Partition Coefficients Between Hexane and Phosphate Buffer
for the Various Phenothiazines of Interest

DRUG	A [a,b] B1	B [b]	A B2	B	A B3	B	A B4	B	A B5	B	A MEAN	B	A	B	CV%
ACEPROMAZINE	10.50	10.00	6.60	5.4	9.00	8.0	6.78	6.0	7.78	8.23	9.13	8.77	9.18	9.21	2.7	13.7
THIORIDAZINE	136	101.64	170	125	170	114	132	58.64	.	.	152	113	58	9.54	11	8.4
CHLORPROMAZINE	148	144	127	163	74	62	138	103	.	.	129	103	48.37	28.93	31.2	28
TRIFLUOPERAZINE	.	472	.	197	176	145	238	188	145	237	193	197	32	26	94.7	13.1
FLUPHENAZINE	14.28	9.60	16.21	14.25	12.98	20	12.52	7.81	14.72	10.96	14.52	12.62	1.44	4.6	11.55	35.60
MESORIDAZINE	.	0.015	.	0.015	.	.	.	0.004	.	0.012	.	0.014	0.0016	0.0016	.	10.4
PROMAZINE	357.00	71	437	84.26	275	92.86	465	82.93	534	95.63	405	85.39	80.03	8.46	19.76	10.75

[a] Determined by actual measurement of the concentration in the two phases.

[b] Determined according to the formula described in the text.

Table 7: Red Blood Cell Partition Coefficient as a Function of Lipophilicity and Concentration for the Phenothiazines of Interest

DRUG	CONC (ng/ml)	A^b	P^c	DET^d	SE^f A	C	D	CV A	C	D	n A	C	D
ACETPROMAZINE L=4.13^a	300	5.57	6.08	9.72	0.23	0.22	0.57	16.44	13.9	16.72	8	7	8
	500	3.83	4.48	5.95	0.26	0.20	0.37	13.6	13.1	17.67	8	8	8
	1000	4.39	5.11	6.44	0.25	0.13	0.18	6.17	10.29	8.1	8	8	8
	NB(1000)	1.26	1.31	—	0.17	0.2	—	29.59	44.09	—	8	8	—
FLUPHENAZINE L=14.92	300	3.67	4.55	4.08	0.41	0.52	0.49	26	20	20	6	6	6
	500	3.47	3.99	7.43	0.19	.24	0.24	13.5	13.36	11.14	5	5	5
	1000	3.17	4.61	9.45	1.03	0.01	1.32	64	33	33	4	4	5
	NB(333)	1.39	3.63	1.44	.089	0.3	005	0.7	15.19	1.13	8	8	0
TRICLOROAZINE L=133	300	4.66	5.61	8.9	0.49	0.44	1.44	23.58	25.6	34.24	8	9	8
	500	3.63	6.63	12.12	0.31	0.65	2.8	18.25	16.77	44	4	3	4
	1000	5.77	6.3	11.79	0.31	0.23	0.53	9.63	9.76	12.01	7	7	7
	NB(1000)	0.38	0.28	0.47	0.03	0.03	0.11	24.6	25.17	23.8	8	8	0
TRIFLUOPROMAZINE L=193	300	5.53	6.02	7.74	—	—	—	—	—	—	2	2	2
	500	4.66	5.39	6.24	0.41	0.5	0.28	17.8	18.5	26.23	4	4	3
	1000	7.48	9.78	11.19	0.71	0.34	1.53	25.3	9.2	27.3	7	7	4
	NB(1000)	1.57	1.7	3.77	0.06	0.08	0.18	10	13	13.5	8	8	0
PROMAZINE L=45	300	5.66	6.38	8.36	0.3	0.28	0.17	13.66	10.77	8.52	8	7	6
	1000	5.95	6.53	7.21	0.19	0.18	0.29	9.17	6.53	6.53	8	8	8
	NB(1000)	1.26	1.41	1.29	0.07	0.11	0.1	13.19	19.74	23.52	6	7	6
MESORIDAZINE L=0.076	5000	3.51	2.70	6.15	0.19	0.11	0.54	9.99	8.02	21.62	6	5	6
	1000	2.36	2.62	3.72	0.09	0.14	0.16	9.33	11.2	10.25	6	6	6
	NB(1000)	0.62	0.51	1.26	0.03	0.04	0.16	14.3	21.6	28.6	8	8	8

^{a}Lipophilicity as measured by the partition coefficient between hexane and phosphate buffer pH 7.4.

^{b}Determined by the actual measurement of both the supernatant and RBC phase.

^{c}Red blood cell partition coefficient.

^{d}Corrected for the presence of plasma water in the RBC.

^{e}Calculated according to the formula described in the text.

^{f}Standard error

^{g}Coefficient of variation

^{h}Number of replicates

TABLE 8: Analysis of Variance for the Concentration Dependency of
the Red Blood Cell Partitioning for the Phenothiazines
Studied

Drug	SOURCE	df	SS	MS	F
Acepromazine	between	2	59.25	29.62	41.13
	within	18	13.04	0.72	
	Total	20			
Fluphenazine	between	2	0.71	0.355	0.11
	within	17	54	3.19	
	total	19			
Trifluoroperazine	between	2	46.71	23.35	2.5
	within	10	93.49	9.35	
	total	12			
Thioridazine	between	2	108.41	54.2	2.22
	within	13	316.3	24.33	
	total	15			

Mesoridazine   tcalc= 0.789 <1
Promazine   tcalc= 0.96 <1

Table 9: Extent of Protein Binding for the Phenothiazines Studied as Determined from their Red Blood Cell Partitioning.

Drug	% bound to proteins	Range[a]
Acepromazine	74	70 - 79
Fluphenazine[b]	67.5	60 -64
Thioridazine	95.5	94.9 -96.16
Trifluoroperazine	82.61	80.94-84
Promazine	78.32	76-80.62

a   The range was calculated as follows:
The lower range was: 1- (Kd+SE)/(D-SE)
The upper range was: 1- (Kd-SE)/(D+SE)
b- The concentration for fluphenazine was 333 ng/ml.

was found to be 75 % bound to plasma proteins at a concentration of 1000 ng/ml. Ballard and coworkers found that for the same concentration range the fraction bound was almost 90 %. This result most probably is not accurate because it means that acepromazine would have a partition coefficient between phosphate buffer pH 7.4 and the red blood cells of over 15 which is very unlikely and very seldomly encountered with any drug. Hu determined the plasma protein binding of promazine by ultracentrifugation and found that only 25 % of the drug was unbound. From our calculations, the free fraction of drug was 22 % (53).

It is notable that these results are of little significance clinically because 1000 ng/ml is too high a concentration and would seldomly be encountered in the clinical practice.

Pharmacokinetics-Pharmacodynamics of Acepromazine in the Horse

The respective acepromazine plasma concentrations for all the horses after administration of intravenous doses of 0.15 mg/kg are presented in Table A-3. Figures 5 to 14 show the fitted plasma time profiles for each horse. The maximum Co concentration ranged from 1701 ng/ml to 67 ng/ml with a mean value of 476 ng/ml.

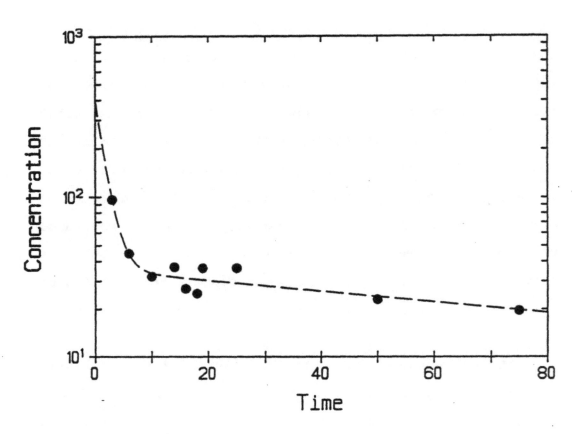

Figure 5: Fitted arterial plasma concentration vs time (min) for horse Letren after an IV administration of 0.15 mg/kg dose of Acepromazine.

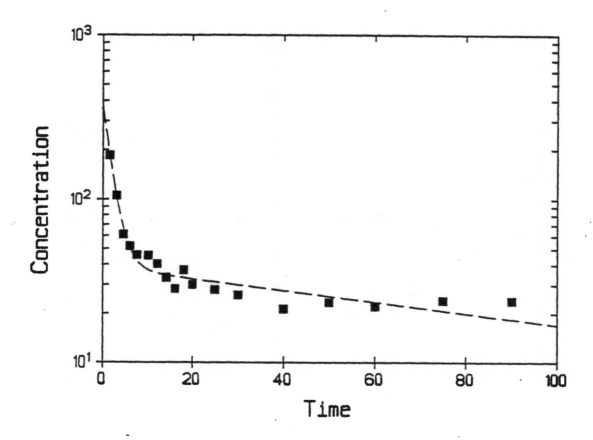

Figure 6: Fitted venous plasma concentration vs time (min) for horse Letren after IV administration of 0.15 mg/kg dose of Acepromazine.

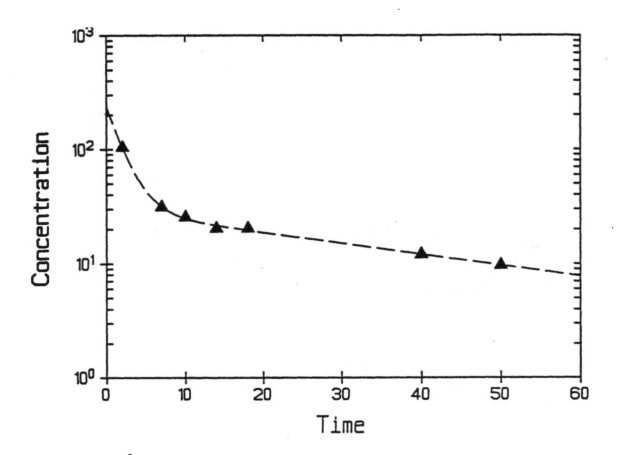

Figure 7: Fitted arterial plasma concentration vs time (min) for horse Dappler Arab after IV administration of 0.15 mg/kg dose of Acepromazine.

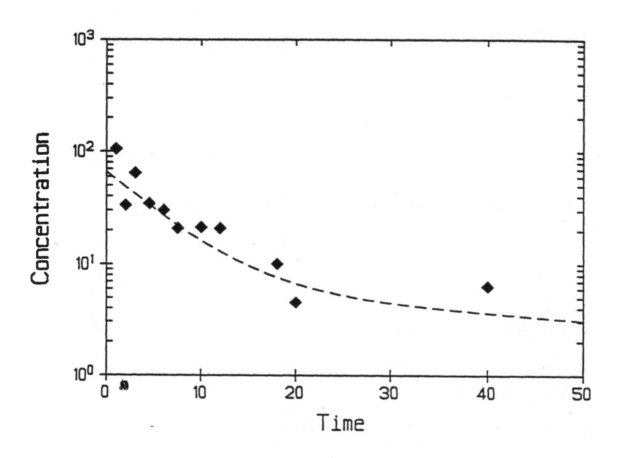

Figure 8: Fitted venous plasma concentration vs time (min) for horse Dappler Arab after IV administration of 0.15 mg/kg dose of Acepromazine.

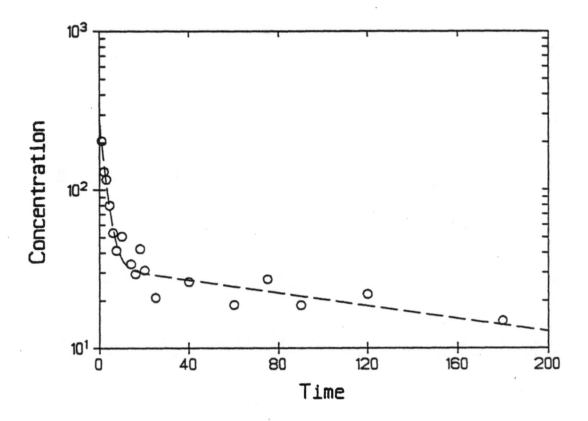

Figure 9: Fitted plasma concentration vs time (min) for horse Chestnut after IV administration pf 0.15 mg/kg dose of Acepromazine.

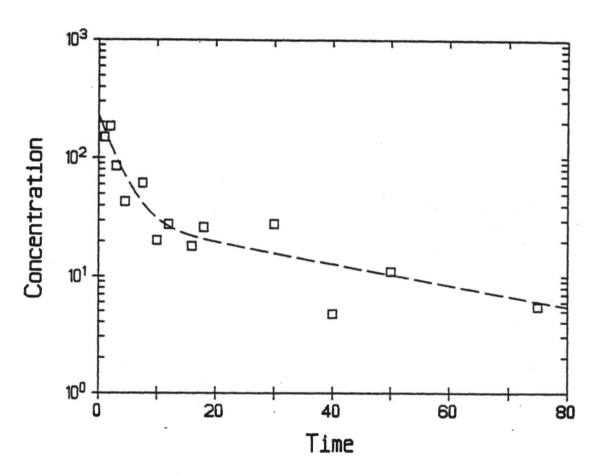

Figure 10: Fitted plasma concentration vs time (min) for horse Sara after IV administration of 0.15 mg/kg dose of Acepromazine.

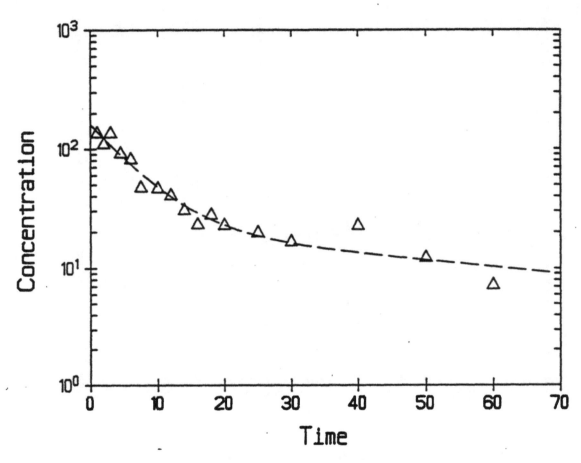

Figure 11: Fitted plasma concentration vs time (min) for horse Juanita after IV administration of 0.15 mg/kg dose of Acepromazine.

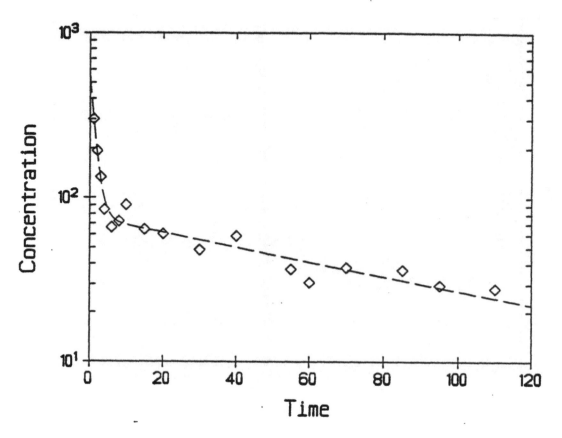

Figure 12: Fitted plasma concentration vs time (min) for horse Raisin after IV administration of 0.15 mg/kg dose of Acepromazine.

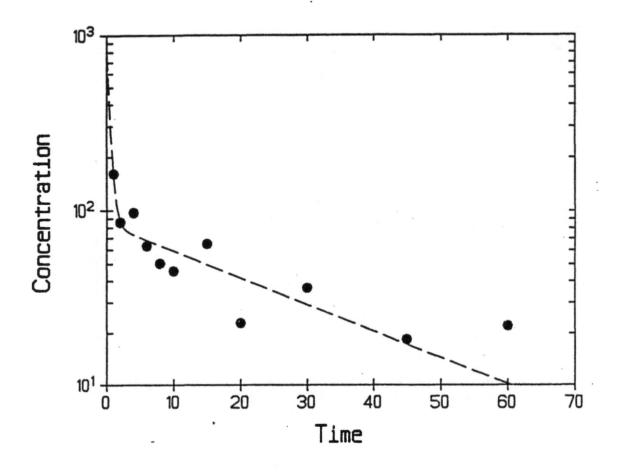

Figure 13: Fitted plasma concentration vs time (min) for horse Roan after IV administration of 0.15 mg/kg dose of Acepromazine.

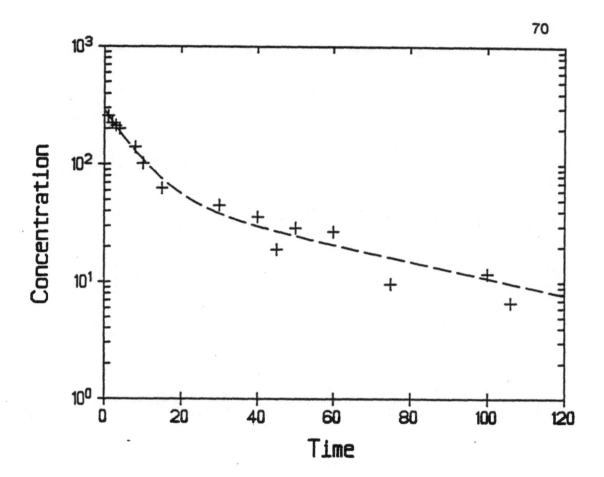

Figure 14: Fitted plasma concentration vs time (min) for horse Roan after IV administration of 0.3 mg/kg dose of Acepromazine.

TABLE 10: Summary of the Pharmacokinetic Parameters for All the Horses After IV Administration of Acepromazine

PARAMETER	LEIREN		JUANITA	CHESTNUT	SARA	DAPPLER		RAISIN	MEAN[a]	SD
	VENOUS	ARTERIAL				VENOUS	ARTERIAL			
Dose(mg)	65	65	82	58	69	58	58	76	66.4	8.86
α(1/min)	0.533	0.59	0.15	0.37	0.32	0.49	0.17	0.72	0.756	0.946
β(1/min)	0.008	0.007	0.013	0.004	0.017	0.022	0.011	0.010	0.014	0.01
a(ng/ml)	327.37	365.66	139.33	236.02	199.49	205.25	61.15	470.06	435.5	496.8
b(ng/ml)	38.82	35.38	21.95	32.51	27.2	29.19	6.08	76.11	41.14	27.08
$t_{\frac{1}{2}}\alpha$(min)	1.30	1.17	4.43	1.88	2.15	1.4	3.97	0.96	2.13	1.434
$t_{\frac{1}{2}}\beta$(min)	81.67	90.29	51.75	148.55	39.45	31.55	59.43	67.63	66.75	38.24
CO(ng/ml)	366.2	401.04	161.28	268.53	226.7	234.44	67.24	546.17	476.77	519.57
AUC(ng/ml/min)	5187	5228.2	2529.3	7608.4	2169.2	1744.1	872.77	8077.7	4188	2601.57
AUMC	540100	601450	128050	1495200	90044	61317	46759	725540	441333	495847
MRT(min)	104.12	115.04	50.62	196.51	41.51	35.15	53.57	89.82	79.76	54.3
Vdss(l)	1303	1430	1621	1497	1320	1169	2559	834	1382	158
Vdss/kg(l)	3.03	3.33	3.0	3.85	2.87	3.0	6.57	1.64	3.15	0.35
Vdpss(l)	1566	1776	2463	1906	1871	1512	6041	928	1863	338
Vdpss/kg(l)	3.65	4.14	4.53	4.9	4.06	3.88	15.52	1.82	4.2	0.45
Vdcc(l)	177.5	162	503	216	304	248	865	137	290	114
Vdcc/kg(l)	0.413	0.377	0.92	0.55	0.66	0.637	2.22	0.27	0.636	0.166
Cltot(ml/min)	12531	12433	32028	7623	31808	33256	66455	9285	23449	11039
Cltot/kg(ml/min)	29.2	28.98	59.01	19.60	69.14	85.49	170.83	18,24	52.49	24.62

[a]averages were calculated for the venous plasma samples without including Raisin

71

Table 11: Confidence Intervals for the Distribution and Elimination
Rate Constants After IV Administration in the Horse

HORSE	ALPHA	SD	95%CI	BETA	SD	95%CI
LEIREN (venous)	0.533	0.472	0.442,0.625	0.00848	0.0022	0.0037,0.013272
LEIREN (arterial)	0.59	0.218	0.055,1.12	0.00767	0.00328	-0.00035,0.0157
JUANITA	0.156	0.0494	0.0496,0.263	0.0133	0.289	-0.049231,0.076
CHESTNUT	0.368	0.0479	0.266,0.4715	0.00466	0.00158	0.00125,0.00807
SARA	0.3212	0.163	-0.048,0.6911	0.0175	0.040	-0.0733,0.108
DAPPLER (arterial)	0.494	0.0451	0.35,0.637	0.0219	0.0023	0.0146,0.0292
DAPPLER (venous)	0.174	0.1289	-0.13,0.4792	0.0116	0.069	-0.15236,0.17568
RAISIN	0.722	0.076	0.577,0.886	0.0102	0.002	0.00586,0.014637

The plasma concentration time profile for all the horses after administration of 0.15 mg /kg doses of acepromazine was fitted best to a two compartment open body model. Acepromazine pharmacokinetic parameters obtained by fitting a two compartment model are summarized in Table 10. The distribution phase with values ranging from 0.13 min -1 to 3.03 min-1 i.e. half-life from 0.23 to 4.43 min , indicated the existence of a relatively fast distribution into a shallow compartment after the drug entered the systemic blood stream. The mean terminal half-life, at 67 +/- 38 min, ranging from 18 to 148 min showed larger variation and relatively slower elimination from the body. The confidence intervals for both rate constants are presented in Table 11. Due to the large variation in the values one can only estimate the magnitude of the rate constants and the half lives. The volume of distribution of the central compartment ranged from 137 l to 503 l with a mean value of 290 liters. These values are much larger than the volume of blood in the horse (70 ml/Kg of body weight) indicating that acepromazine is widely distributed in the horse. The total clearance of acepromazine in the horse after IV administration was found to be 23.5 +/-11 l/min (52.49+/-24.62 ml/min/kg). This value was determined by taking the ratio of the dose divided by the area under the curve up to time infinity. This total clearance value is not significantly differeny than the cardiac output in the horse which is around 18 l/min (54) indicating that this drug does not undergo any non flow dependent metabolism. Therefore the plasma clearance or metabolism contribution to the total clearance is negligible. However, the contribution of each organ to the total clearance is unknown since the rena clearance of acepromazine could not be determined.

The only other study about the pharmacokinetics of acepromazine in the horse was done by Ballard and Coworkers where they administered 0.3 mg/kg. They obtained an alpha phase half life of 4.2 min and an elimination half life of 185 min. Both these values are almost triple that obtained in the present work. This might be due to the fact that they gave a dose double the present dose. The difference might also be due to the fact that the analytical method might be different enabling us to measure lower concentration. Another difference might be that their reported value was not be the terminal phase but a value of a second compartment that they were able to see because of their higher dose. Interestingly enough, the values for the total clearance agree well with each other, their value was 25 l/min while the one obtained here was 23.5 l/min even though the dose in this study was half of theirs. This strongly suggests that the pharmacokinetics of acepromazine in the horse behave in a linear fashion.

It is notable that even though horse Letren sufferred from a mitral valve insufficiency in its heart affecting somewhat its cardiac output. Although showing no sign of frank cardiac failure, this deficiency did not affect the disposition of acepromazine in this horse since the pharmacokinetic parameters obtained from this horse were very similar to what was obtained with other horses. Horse Letren but not horse Dappler Arab showed the same pharmacokinetic profile when venous and arterial plasma concentrations were plotted versus time. All the pharmacokinetic parameters were the same for the horse Letren but not for horse Dappler Arab (refer to Table 8). The terminal half life for horse Letren was 82 min for the venous plasma levels and 90 min for the arterial samples. As for horse Dappler Arab, the terminal half life was 32 and 59 min for the venous and arterial samples respectively. This is not to say that there were no differences between the venous and arterial plasma samples. For the first three minutes, the venous plasma samples (the drug was injected into the venous side) showed higher concentrations of drug than the arterial samples taken at the same time points. After this initial time of three minutes the plasma concentrations were the same on either side indicating that the drug had been redistributed and been circulated all over the body and thus reached equilibrium between the two sides.

PHARMACODYNAMIC EFFECTS OF ACEPROMAZINE IN THE HORSE

A-Effect on the Equine Hematocrit

Table A-8 summarizes the hematocrit values as a function of time for all the five horses that were given 0.15 mg/Kg. A plot of the hematocrit values vs time is given in Figure 15. It can be seen that at this dose level, acepromazine has a profound effect on the hematocrit. In all the horses studied the hematocrit dropped by more than 20 %. This drop in hematocrit was not immediate but was gradual and reached the lowest value after six hours. This is not to say that the biggest effect on the hematocrit occurred at six hours, the study was stopped at this time and it is possible that a further reduction might have occurred after this time period. Also it was not possible to determine how long this reduction might have lasted. These results agree very well with other investigators who

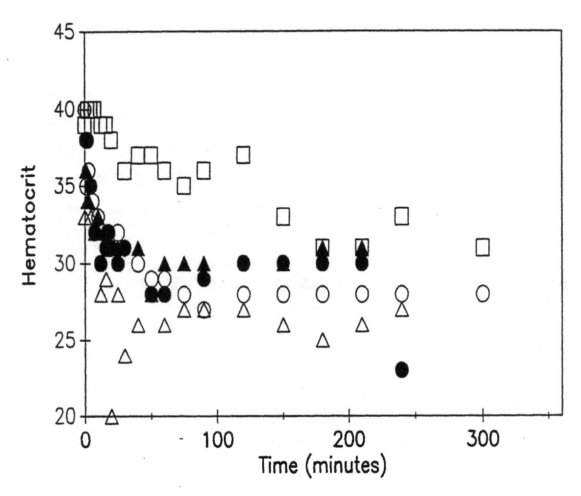

Figure 15: Plot of hematocrit vs time for all 5 horses after
IV administration of 0.15 mg/kg dose of Acepromazine. (O)
Dappler; (●) Juanita; (△) Sara; (▲) Chestnut;
(□) Letren.

found that the duration and not the degree of the decrease in the hematocrit was dose related. Parry and Anderson found that the hematocrit returned to its control value twenty one hours after acepromazine administration.

The mechanism of action of this decrease is thought to be due to the alpha-adrenolytic activity of acepromazine together with a depression of the vasomotor centre causing splenic relaxation with consequent erythrocyte sequestration causing a drop in the hematocrit values. The fact that this decrease is not dose dependent might be due to the fact that it is dependent on the splenic storage capacity.

B-Cardiovacular and Hemodynamic Effect of Acepromazine

A summary of the systolic, diastolic and mean blood pressure as a function of time are given in Table A-4 while the heart rates for all the horses after acepromazine administration are given in Table A-5. Figure 16, 17 and 18 show the plot of the systolic, diastolic and mean blood pressure as a function of time while Figure 19 show the plot of the heart rate as a function of time for all the horses given 0,15 mg/kg of acepromazine. Table A-7 summarizes the blood gases as a function of time for the five horses studied.

In all the horses studied (except for horse Letren) there was a marked decrease in systolic blood pressure. As seen with the hematocrit, this drop in systolic blood pressure was not sudden but was gradual and reached its maximum decrease between 60 and 90 minutes post administration of the acepromazine dose. In four out the five horses, the systolic blood pressure dropped from a value of around 140 mm of Hg to values around 100 in a time period of approximately 100 minutes. These values remained depressed even after the elapse of up to six hours. Horse Letren did not show any marked changes in its systolic blood pressure. This might be due to the fact that Letren sufferred already from some hemodynamic problems and thus would not be expected to react normally to the pharmacological actions of acepromazine.

The same trend was also observed for both the diastolic and mean blood pressure. They exhibited the same pattern as was observed with the systolic blood pressure. The drop was gradual over a certain period of time and its maximal decrease at about the same time. Again in horse Letren the changes in these blood pressures were not as obvious as with the other horses. This decrease in blood pressure might be due to a direct effect on the heart and

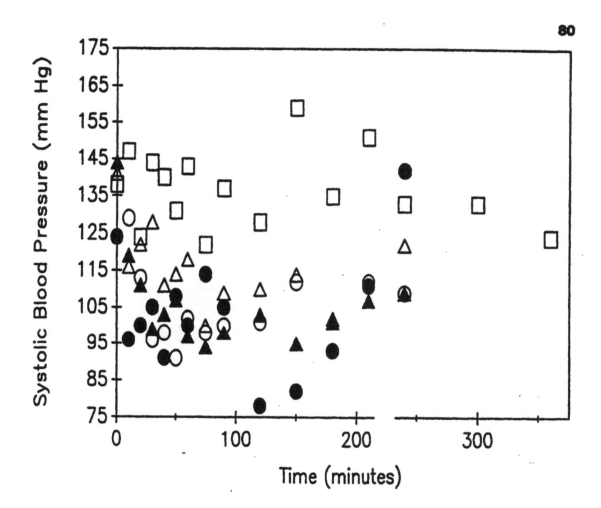

Figure 16: Plot of the systolic blood pressure (mm HG) vs time (minutes) for all 5 hourses after IV administration of 0.15 mg/kg dose of acepromazine. (○) Dappler; (●) Juanita; (△) Sara; (▲) Chestnut; (□) Letren.

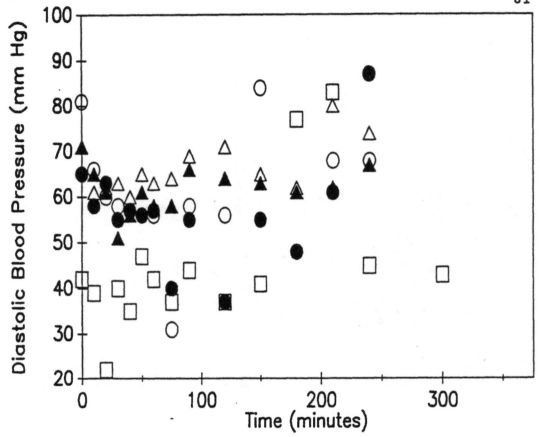

Figure 17: Plot of the diastolic blood pressure (mm Hg) vs time for all 5 horses after IV administration of 0.15mg/kg dose of Acepromazine. (O) Dappler; (●) Juanita; (△) Sara; (▲) Chestnut; (□) Letren.

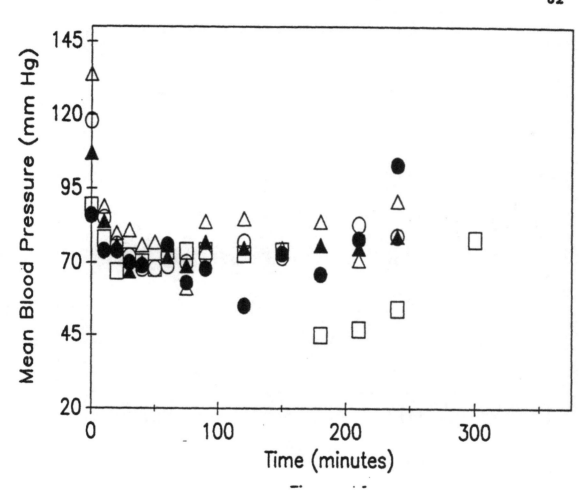

Figure 18: Plot of the mean blood pressure for all 5 horses after IV administration of 0.15 mg/kg dose of Acepromazine. (O) Dappler; (●) Juanita; (△) Sara; (▲) Chestnut; (□) Letren.

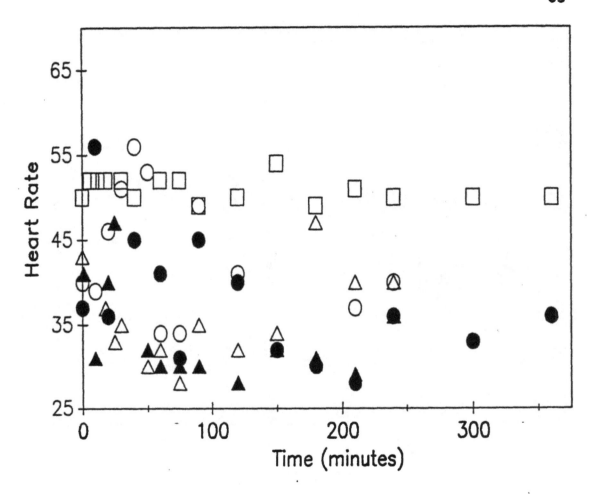

Figure 19: Plot of the heart rate vs time for all 5 horses
after IV administration of 0.15 mg/kg dose of Acepromazine.
(O) Dappler; (●) Juanita; (△) Sara; (▲) Chestnut;
(□) Letren.

blood vessels and also indirect ones through actions on CNS and autonomic reflexes. However, alpha adrenergic blockade on the blood vessels might be the primary cause for this decrease. Thus because of this induced hypotension reflex tachycardia is expected. However, if we look at Figure 19, it can be seen that the heart rate was also decreased from an average value of 40 to 42 down to a value around 28. Again as was observed with other pharmacological actions, this decrease in heart rate was gradual and reached a maximum around 100 minutes. This decrease in heart rate is thought to be due to either a direct adrenergic blocking effect in the heart or due to some sort of centrally mediated action which was much stronger than the reflex tachycardia that was due to the induced hypotension. This is in agreement with the results obtained by other investigators who found an average decrease in heart rates of about 25%

Even though a marked change in blood pressure and a marked decrease in heart rate occurred, this did not have any effect on either the blood gases or the physiological pH. This was most probably due to the fact that the respiration rate (which was not measured in the present study) was not affected by acepromazine. This was contrary to expectation because other phenothiazines including acepromazine are known to cause centrally mediated respiratory depression. The absence of significant changes in arterial carbon dioxide and oxygen tension may reflect a compensatory increase in tidal volume to maintain an appropriate minute alveolar ventilation. It is interesting to note that horse Letren had higher carbon dioxide tension and lower pH values due to the fact that this horse was suffering from cardiac insufficiency.

C-CNS AND SEDATIVE EFFECTS OF ACEPROMAZINE IN THE HORSE

The different CNS parameters measured as a function of time are summarized in Table A-6. It can be seen that among all the CNS parameters measured the reaction to noise was the least sensitive and useful in evaluating the sedative and CNS effects of acepromazine. Figures 20 to 23 show the degree of eyelid droop, the reaction to the pinprick test, the head carriage and the extent of movement respectively as a function of time. As can be seen from these plots, the most sensitive indicators for the sedative and CNS effects were the head carriage and the eyelid droop. It can be clearly seen that the more sedated the horse is the lower his head carriage would be. Naturally, the more sedated the

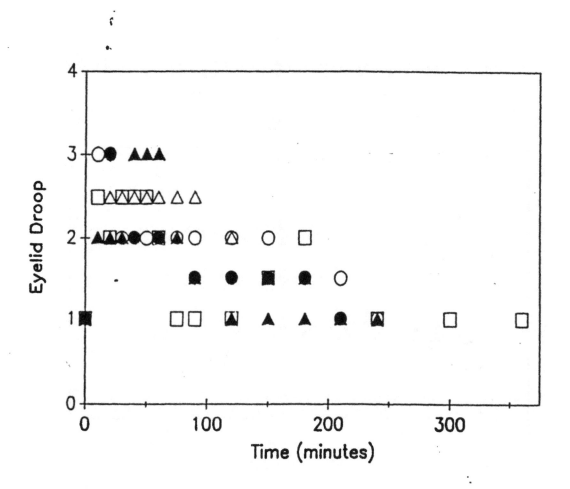

Figure 20: Plot of the degree of eyelid droop vs time for all 5 horses after IV administration of 0.15 mg/kg dose of Acepromazine. (O) Dappler; (●) Juanita; (△) Sara; (▲) Chestnut; (□) Letren.

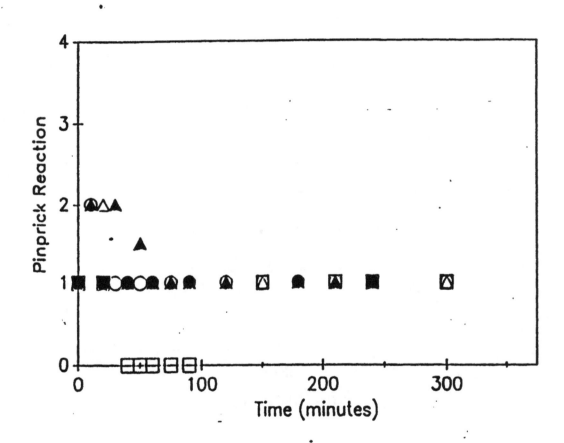

Figure 21: Plot of the reaction to the pin prick test vs time for all 5 horses after IV administration of 0.15 mg/kg dose of Acepromazine. (O) Dappler; (●) Juanita; (△) Sara; (▲) Chestnut; (□) Letren.

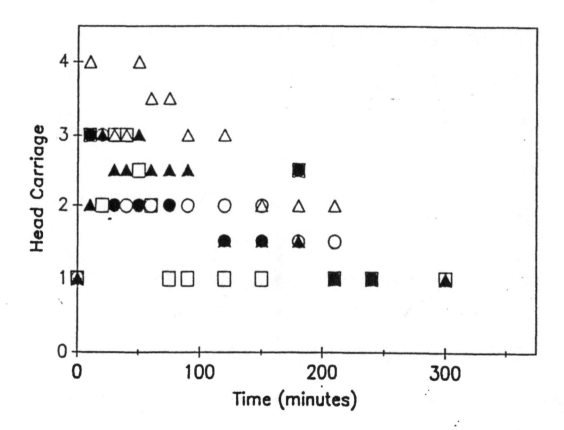

Figure 22: Plot of the head carriage vs time for all 5 horses after IV administration of 0.15 mg/kg dose of Acepromazine. (O) Dappler; (●) Juanita; (△) Sara; (▲) Chestnut; (□) Letren·

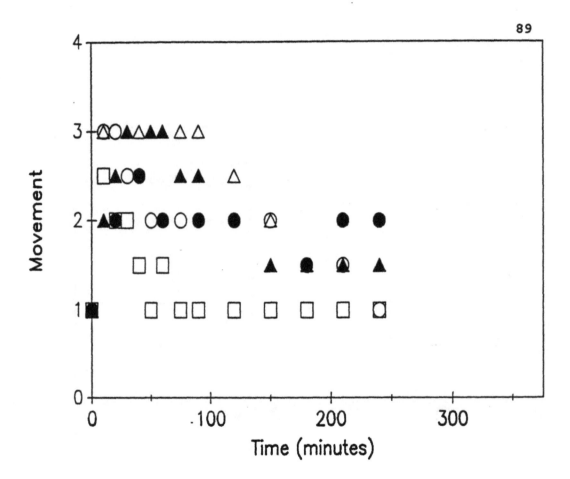

Figure 23: Plot of the extent of movement vs time for all 5 horses after IV administration of 0.15 mg/kg dose of Acepromazine. (O) Dappler; (●) Juanita; (△) Sara; (▲) Chestnut;(□) Letren.

horse is the less movement he is going to exhibit as can be seen from Figure 23. A clear trend is obvious in all the plots of these sedative effects is that the peak or maximum effect occurs at a much faster time than the cardiovascular effects and last longer in duration. The peak effects occur at around 10 to 20 minutes compared to the peak hypotension occuring at around 100 minutes and usually last for up to 150 minutes post acepromazine administration. The onset of action is much faster and the recovery from the sedation occurs quite quickly. These sedative and CNS effects are thought to be centrally mediated and is thought to be due to the antagonism of dopamine mediated synaptic transmission.

It is to note that in the only male horse in the study (horse Letren) pronounced priapism occurred and lasted until the study was completed. The duration of this priapism was not determined because the horse was not monitored after the six hour period the time for the last plasma collection. This priapism is well documented in the literature and is most probably due to the alpha adrenergic blocking actions of acepromazine resulting in paralysis of the retractor muscle of the penis.

D-PHARMACODYNAMIC-PHARMACOKINETIC CORRELATION

None of the observed pharmacodynamic parameters correlated well with the plasma levels of acepromazine. The peak effects occurred at a much later time while the concentration of acepromazine was decreasing. This might be due to the fact that these pharmacological effects are mediated by an active metabolite of acepromazine and thus there is a lag time for the formation of sufficient amounts of metabolites to exert a noticeable pharmacological effects or it might be due to the fact that the receptors are located in a deep compartment and thus it takes some time for the drug to reach sufficient concentrations in the biophase.

Additionally, the onset of the sedative and CNS effects seem to be faster than the cardiovascular effects might be due to the fact that the site for the receptors might be in a shallow compartment which is more accessible for the drug. The other reason might be due to the fact that it takes a much longer time to affect the cardiovascular system due to the fact that there are many other hemodynamic factors that will control all these pharmacodynamic parameters.

PHARMACOKINETICS OF ACEPROMAZINE IN THE CAT

The plasma concentration as a function of time for all the four cats after intravenous administration of a 0.3 mg/kg dose are summarized in Table A-9. Figure 24 to Figure 27 show the fitted plasma concentrations vs time for the respective cats.

The various pharmacokinetic parameters obtained from this study are summarized in Table 12. Table 13 gives the confidence intervals for the rate constants obtained after IV administration of the drug. The extrapolated time 0 concentration had a mean value of 1175 +/-1349. These values ranged from a low of 129 ng/ml to a maximal value of 3490 ng/ml which seemed unexpectedly high. These results show a great deal of variabilty that might be due to either a difference in the distribution of the drug or due to a big difference in the volume of the central compartment. The volume of the central compartment ranged from 0.43 to 8.6 liters with a mean value of 3.52 +/- 3.11 liters. This value is much larger than the plasma volume which is 41 ml/kg of body weight or the blood volume which is 55 ml/kg. This means that acepromazine is very widely distributed in the body and that the central compartment is not confined to the blood or plasma. The volume of distribution at steady

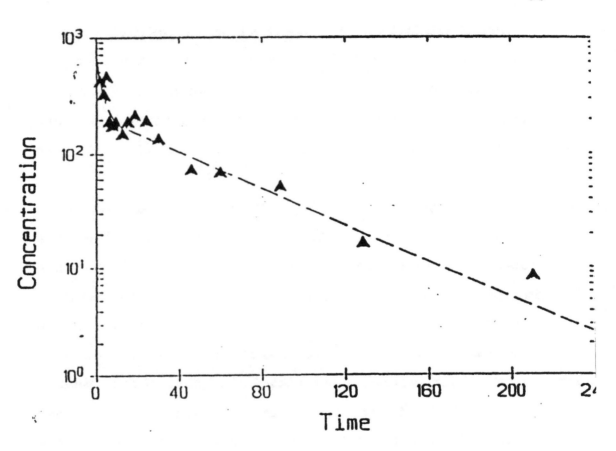

Figure 24: Plot of fitted plasma concentration vs time (min) for cat Green 1, after IV administration of 0.3 mg/kg dose of Acepromazine

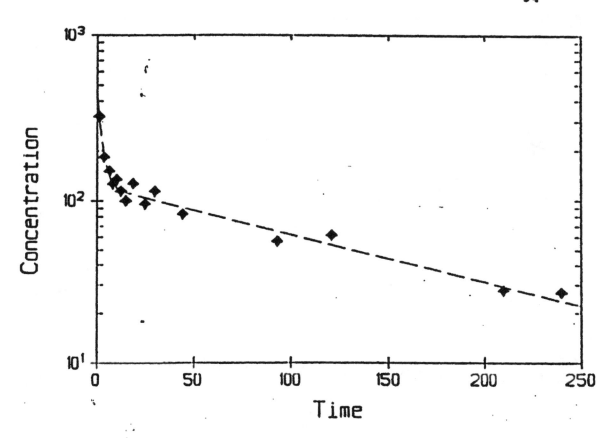

Figure 25: Plot of the fitted plasma concentration vst time (min) for cat Red 1, after IV administration of 0.3 mg/kg dose of Acepromazine

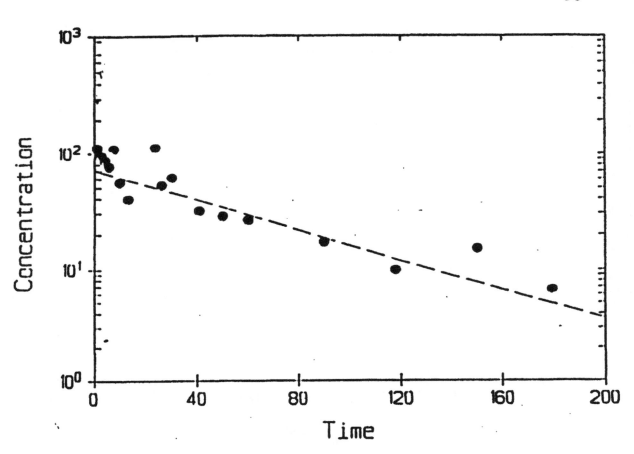

Figure 26: Plot of the fitted plasma concentration vs time (min) for cat Green 2, after IV administration of 0.3 mg/kg dose of Acepromazine

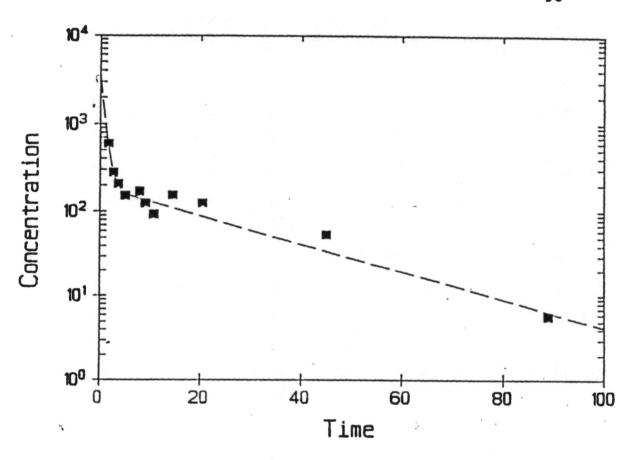

Figure 27: Plot of the fitted plasma concentration vs time (min) for cat Red 2, after IV administration of 0.3 mg/kg of Acepromazine

TABLE 12: Summary of the Pharmacokinetic Parameters After IV
Administration of a 0.3 mg/kg Dose of Acepromazine
in the 4 Cats.

PARAMETER	GREEN1	RED1	GREEN2	RED2	MEAN	SD
Dose(mg)	1.11	1.44	1.11	1.53	1.30	0.19
α(1/min)	0.417	0.405	0.207	1.302	0.583	0.423
β(1/min)	0.018	0.006	0.012	0.038	0.018	0.012
a(ng/ml)	432	307.3	76.94	3300	1029	1317.3
b(ng/ml)	220.21	121.54	53	189.73	146.12	64.55
$t_{\frac{1}{2}} \alpha$ (min)	1.66	1.71	3.33	0.532	1.808	0.997
$t_{\frac{1}{2}} \beta$ (min)	37.11	111.71	57.62	18.2	56.16	34.97
CO (ng/ml)	652.17	428.84	129	3490	1175	1349
AUC(ng/mlmin)	12825	20347	4773.2	7514.3	11365	5939
AUMC	633740	3158900	367800	132710	1073287	1217105
MRT(min)	49.14	155	77.05	17.66	74.7	50.89
Vdss(l)	4.2	10.97	17.87	3.55	9.15	5.81
Vdss/kg(l)	1.13	2.28	4.83	0.70	2.23	1.6
Vdpss(l)	4.8	11.79	19.33	5.28	10.3	5.9
Vdpss/kg(l)	1.3	2.45	5.22	1.03	2.5	1.65
Vdcc(l)	1.7	3.35	8.6	0.43	3.52	3.11
Vdcc/kg(l)	0.46	0.70	2.32	0.084	0.89	0.85
Cltot(ml/min)	86.55	70.77	232	201	147.58	70
Cltot/kg(ml/min)	23.39	14.74	62.70	46.73	36.89	18.95

TABLE 13: Confidence Interval for the Distribution and Elimination Rate Constants
After IV Administration in the Cat.

CAT	ALPHA	SD	95%CI	BETA	SD	95%CI
GREEN1	0.471	0.274	-0.1799, 1.0148	0.0186	0.0042	0.0094, 0.0279
RED1	0.4049	0.0911	0.208, 0.601	0.0062	0.00066	0.00477, 0.00763
GREEN2	0.20766	0.12767	-0.0705, 0.485	0.012	0.0018133	0.00807, 0.015980
RED2	1.302	0.659	-0.25732, 2.863	0.038091	0.00329	0.0302, 0.04588

state was 9.15 +/-5.81.   The values ranged from a low of 3.55 to a high value of 17.87 liters.

The plasma concentration following intravenous administration of 0.3 mg/kg of acepromazine was best fitted to an open two compartment body model. Similarly to what was obtained with the horses, the distribution phase rate constants ranged from 0.207 to 1.3 min-1 with a mean value of 0.583, ie half life values from 0.532 to 3.33 minutes, indicating the existence of a relatively fast distribution into a shallow compartment after the drug entered the systemic blood stream. The mean terminal half-life , 56 +/- 35 minutes, range 18.2 to 112 minutes showed longer variation and relatively slow elimination from the body. This is in agreement with the results obtained with the horse studies (alpha phase half-life of 2.13 min and a terminal half-life of 66 min).   Even the volume of distribution of the central compartment were very similar on a l/Kg basis. In the horse it was around one l/Kg while in the cat it was around 1.2 l/Kg strongly suggesting that there is no species difference in either the disposition or the distribution of acepromazine in the horse and the cat. The total clearance of acepromazine in the cat was determined to be 147.58 ml/min +/-70 (range 70 to 232 ml/min).

Unfortunately, there are no pharmacokinetic studies in the cat reported in the literature, therefore no comparison or inferences on the validity of the results obtained could be drawn.

Bioavailabilty of Acepromazine after Oral, Subcutaneous and Intramuscular administration

Table A-10, A-11, A-12 summarize the plasma concentrations after oral administration of 10 mg tablets of acepromazine and SC and IM administration of 0.3 mg/kg doses. Figure 28 depicts the plasma concentrations as a function of time for all the three cats that showed any plasma level after oral administration. Table 14 summarizes the most important pharmacokinetic parameters.

As can be seen the plasma levels obtained after oral administration of a 10 mg tablet of acepromazine were much lower than those obtained with the IV route even though the dose was almost 10 times higher. In cat Red 2 no acepromazine concentrations were detectable in the plasma. In all the other 3 cats the bioavailabilty was poor and never exceeded 50 %. The bioavailable fraction of the drug that reached the systemic circulation intact ranged from 12 to 48 %. It is interesting to note that the plasma levels obtained after oral administration were very erratic and could not be adequately fitted to any pharmacokinetic model. The poor bioavailability of acepromazine might be due to poor absorption from the gastrointestinal tract, or most probably, a very high first-pass effect. The drug would be extensively metabolized before it even reaches the systemic circulation. Phenothiazines are well known to undergo an extensive first pass effect and thus will show a very erratic plasma profile after oral administration.

The maximum plasma concentration obtained was consistent in the three cats. The Cpmax ranged from 73 to 98 ng/ml. However, the time to reach maximum concentration was widely different in the three cats. The Tmax ranged from 41 to 163 minutes. This large variation in the time to reach peak concentrations might be due to big differences in the rate of absorption in the three cats. The absorption rate constants that were obtained when trying to fit data to a model with first order absorption, were very close to the values of the terminal phase. Therefore the absorption half lives that were obtained are hybrid rate constant because elimination is occurring at a rate almost equal to the absorption rate and thus the values that were obtained have no real meaning or significance. Thus the need to use the Loo-Riegelman method for estimating the fraction of the absorbable or the fraction of the absorbable drug remaining to be absorbed as a function of time. The plot of the natural logarithm of the fraction of absorbable drug remaining to be absorbed as a function of time for all the three cats that showed any acepromazine plasma is presented in Figures 31 and 32. It can be seen that for cats green 2 and Red 1 the ln of the fraction remaining to be absorbed vs time gave a straight line signifying that acepromazine absorption was a first order process. In cat Green 1 , the fit was not as good signifying that the absorption process was not typically first order and not typically zero order but most probably an erratic process that did not follow any pattern or model. The absorption rate constants that were obtained using these Loo-Riegelman plots were 0.01047 for cat Green 1,0.00932 for cat Green 2 and 0.0215 for cat Red 1 corresponding to half-life values for the absorption phase of 66, 74 and 32 minutes respectively. These results show that the interindividual variability from one cat to the other was very small. This is somewhat surprising because most phenothiazines show a great variability and difference in their plasma concentrations and pharmacokinetic parameters.

The pharmacokinetics of acepromazine after oral

administration can be best described as exhibiting an almost flip-flop since the absorption rate constants and the elimination rate constants are very close to each other and thus absorption of the drug would be still occurring at the end the time profile. Additionally, since the absorption is occurring at a relatively slow rate, the distribution phase will not be seen and a vanishing exponential phenomenon would occur. Actually, when the oral plasma concentrations are plotted versus time no rapid distribution phase is observed.

Bioavailability of Acepromazine after SC and IM Administration in the Cat

The plasma concentration after subcutaneous and intramuscular administration of the 0.3 mg/kg dose in the four cats studied are presented in Table A-11 and A-12 respectively. Figure 29 depicts the plot of the plasma concentration as a function of time after subcutaneous administration while Figure 30 gives he profile for the plasma concentrations after intramuscular administration. Table 14 and 15 summarize the pharmacokinetic parameters of interest for the subcutaneous and intramuscular route repectively.

TABLE 14: Summary of the Pharmacokinetic Parameters After Oral
Administration of 10 mg Tablet of Acepromazine to Cats.   104

PARAMETER	GREEN1	RED1	GREEN2
AUC	35784	16783	15928
Lag Time(min)	31.17	17	0
Cpmax (ng/ml)	98.46	77.35	72
Tmax (min)	163.38	97.54	41.45
f	0.301	0.123	0.48

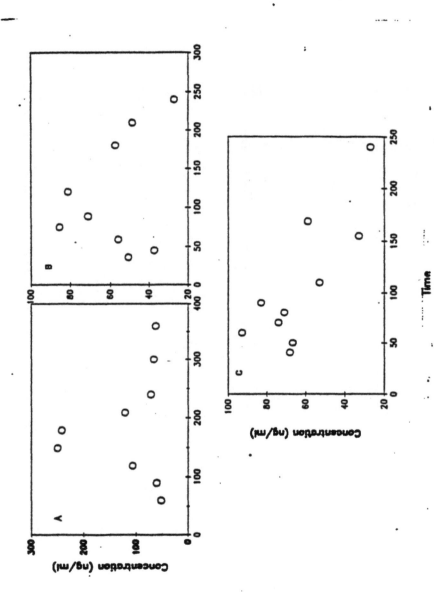

Figure 28: Plot of plasma concentration after an oral
administration of 10 mg of Acepromazine, Table 1, to: Cat Green
1 (Panel A); Cat Red 1 (Panel B); Cat Green 2 (Panel C).

From the above plots it is clear that the intramuscular route gives much higher plasma concentrations than either the oral or subcutaneous route. In the two cats the maximum plasma concentration was around 330 ng/ml which was very comparable to the IV maximal concentration and it occurred relatively rapidly. In cat Green 1 the tmax was 0 and in cat Red 1 it was only 22 min. However with the subcutaneous route the maximum concentration was much more fluctuating and from a value of 38 ng/ml to a high of 184 ng/ml. Also the time to reach this maximum concentration was longer for the subcutaneous route. The tmax ranged from a relatively fast time of 0 minutes to 62 minutes. The bioavailability was much lower after SC administration. It ranged from 0.264 to 0.753 while the values obtained with the IM route was almost equal to 1 and in one cat was even greater than 1. This result is most probably an outlier because it is not physiologically possible to get a bioavailability value greater than 1. This erroneous result might be due to the fact that the intravenous AUC was smaller than its actual value or it might be due to the fact that the physiology of this specific cat had changed in a way that it altered the pharmacokinetics or the disposition of acepromazine giving higher plasma levels than the intravenous route.

It is very interesting to note that the plasma profile was very different from one cat to the other. In three of the four cats, there was a clear relatively fast absorption phase followed by an elimination phase. However, the distribution phase was not observable because the absorption was not fast enough compared to the distribution of the drug. The only exception to that was cat Red 1 where there was no absorption phase but the profile was typically biphasic and similar to what was obtained with the intravenous route. The terminal half lives obtained after either SC or IM administration are very close in values with what we obtain after intravenous administration. The terminal half-lives obtained were in the range of 60 to 100 minutes. Thus it can be said that the absorption of acepromazine is much faster and much more complete with either the SC or the IM route when compared to the oral route of administration. The most plausible reason for the fact that in some of the cats no absorption phase is observed is that the absorption occurs at such a fast rate that it could be considered almost instantaneous. This difference in absorption rates might be due to

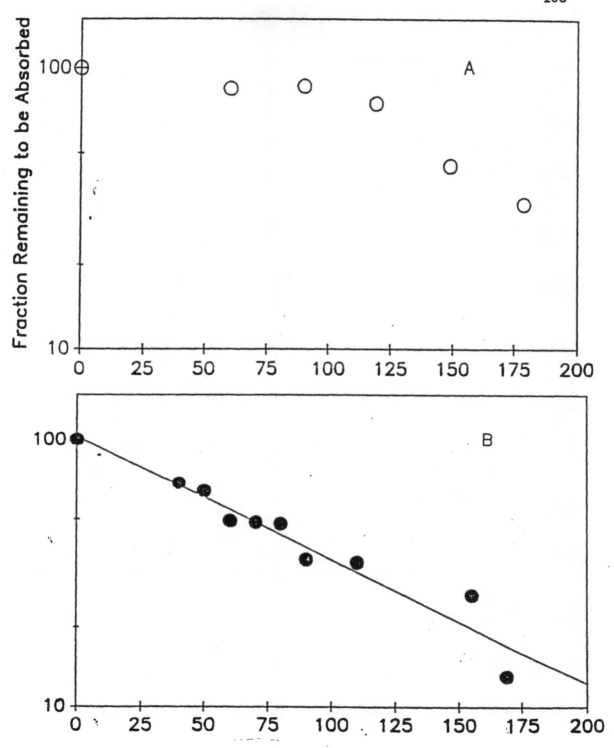

Figure 31:   Plot of the fraction remaining to be absorbed vs time for: Cat Green 1 (Panel A); Cat Green 2 (Panel B).

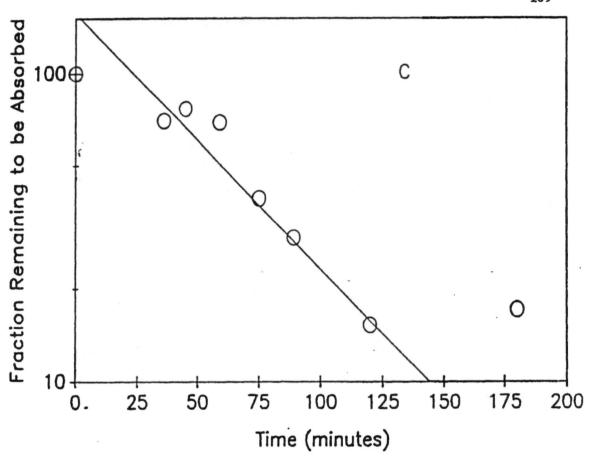

Figure 32:   Plot of the fraction remaining to be absorbed vs
time for Cat Red 1.

interindividual variability or differences in the blood perfusion at the site of administration of the drug.

Effect of Acepromazine on the Hematocrit in the Cat

Table A-12 summarizes the hematocrits measured in the cat after administration of acepromazine via the four different routes. It can be seen that the hematocrit decreased tremendously in all the four cats. The hematocrit decreased from a baseline line value of around 30 pre acepromazine administration to a value of less than 20 %. The extent of this decrease was the same in all the cats regardless of the route of administration. This decrease in hematocrit was more pronounced than what was seen with the horse studies. The decrease in the hematocrit might be due the action of acepromazine as explained previously for the horses, and also due to the fact that frequent blood samples are been withdrawn from the cat with a very limited volume of its blood due to its small size.

To ascertain for sure whether this decrease was due to the frequent sampling or due to the drug, frequent blood sampling of the same amount and frequency should be performed in control cats without any administration of the drug.

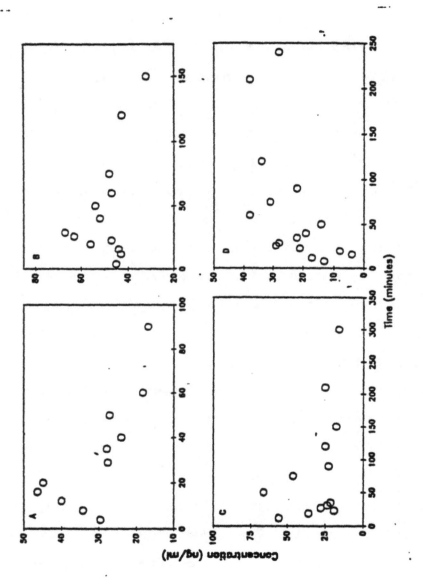

Figure 29: Plot of plasma concentration vs time after a subcutaneous administration of 0.3 mg/kg dose of Acepromazine to: Cat Green 1 (Panel A); Cat Red 1 (Panel B); Cat Green 2 (Panel C); and Cat Red 2 (Panel D).

112

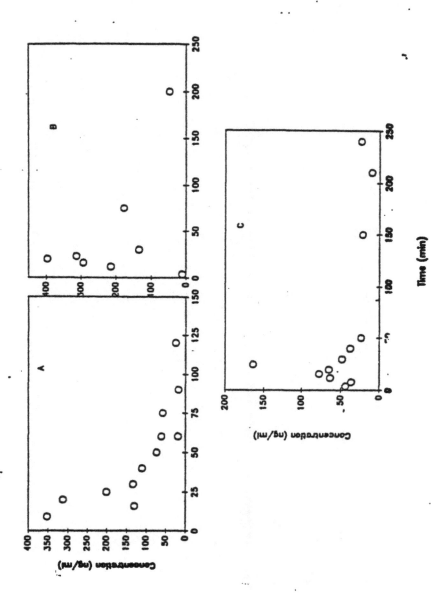

Figure 30: Plot of plasma concentration vs time after an intramuscular administration of 0.3 mg/kg dose of Acepromazine to: Cat Green 1 (Panel A); Cat Red 1 (Panel B); Cat Red 2 (Panel C).

TABLE 15: Summary of the Pharmacokinetic Parameters After Subcutaneous
Administration of a 0.3 mg/kg dose of Acepromazine to the Cat.

PARAMETER	GREEN1	RED1	GREEN2	RED2
AUC	3393.7	15326	11276	2736.4
AUMC	275640	4320500	1707500	315580
MRT(min)	81.22	282	151.41	115.33
$t_{\frac{1}{2}}-1$(min)	54.1	210.29	88.85	46.66
$t_{\frac{1}{2}}-2$(min)	2.181	5.65	30.08	33.28
Cmax (ng/ml)	38	183.55	53.64	38
tmax (min)	10.86	0	42.34	62
lag time (min)	0.305	0	0	5.58
b (ng/ml)	45.3	46.84	113.26	141.75
a(ng/ml)	-45.3	136.71	-73.13	-141.75
K1(1/min)	0.316	0.122	0.023	0.021
K2(1/min)	0.013	0.0033	0.0078	0.015
f	0.264	.753	--	0.36

General Observations

The observed fluctuations in acepromazine plasma levels specially after oral administration could have been caused by assay unreliabilty, variation in absorption rate and/or variation in clearance. The assay reliabilty was fully validated and fluctuation was greater than the assay variance. Another cause for this variabilty might be due to a very erratic dissolution of the tablet resulting in a poor absorption or a very high presystemic metabolism resulting in variances in the overall clearance of the drug from animal to animal.

Additionally, no urine data was obtained. Therefore no information was obtained about the renal clearance of the drug nor the amount of metabolites excreted in the urine. Moreover, the urine data might have picked up a third phase in the disposition of acepromazine because of increased sensitivity because in urine we are dealing with cumulative amounts excreted not concentrations. This might explain the relatively short terminal half-life obtained in both cats and horses. The true terminal half-life might be much longer but because of the extremely low plasma concentrations and the limitations in the sensitivity of the assay, the drug was not detected for a very long time giving rise only to a biphasic profile.

No information about the metabolic fate of acepromazine was obtained from the present studies. Future studies should be performed that will include the monitoring of both the parent drug and its major metabolites in both the plasma and urine. If possible, the metabolites should be administered individually and the pharmacokinetics for each one investigated. This might help explain why the pharmacodynamic effects do not correlate with the plasma levels of the parent compound and why these effects are delayed. This will also help to discover which metabolite is active and which one is not.

Conclusions and Clinical Significance

This work was planned as an investigation of the pharmacokinetic properties of a widely used drug acepromazine about which very little is known. The work involved assay development, studies of certain pharmacokinetically relevant physicochemical properties of acepromazine and a group of pharmacologically and chemically related drugs, studies of red blood cell binding and pharmacokinetic studies in cats and horses.

The following observations were made:

1) All the phenothiazines studied can be measured in biological fluids using liquid chromatography with electrochemical detection without prior derivatization.

2) There was no relationship between the red blood cell partitioning and lipophilicity for all the phenothiazines investigated. Additionally, there was no correlation between concentration and the value of the red blood cell partition coefficient. These phenothiazines were found almost six times more in the red blood cells as compared to the concentration in plasma.

3) In both the cats and horse, the plasma concentration time profile after intravenous administration was biphasic with an alpha distribution half life of 1.8 minutes and an elimination half life of 60 minutes.

4) In the cat, acepromazine showed an erratic absorption profile with a poor bioavailabilty which was very variable from one cat to the other. There is a strong indication of a very high first effect. Subcutaneous and intramuscular doses give higher plasma levels than the oral doses.

5) In both the cat and the horse acepromazine decreased the hematocrit by almost 40 %. In the horse, the systolic, diastolic and mean blood pressure as well as the heart rate were decreased. Additionally, acepromazine had a pronouced sedative effect in all the horses studied. All these pharmacodynamic effects peaked around 100 minutes after administration of the drug.

6) All the pharmacodynamic effects persisted much longer than the drug was detected in the plasma.

Bearing in mind these observations and in view of the relatively short terminal half-life of acepromazine in both the cat and the horse, it is recommended that acepromazine should be administered frequently if a sustained and prolonged sedation is required or desired. It is also important to make sure that the animal in question does not have any cardiac complications or any hypotension since acepromazine as was seen from the results of the present studies have strong hypotensive properties.

As for the route of administration the intravenous route will give the fastest onset of action. However, the results would seem to suggest that the intramuscular route would be better than the subcutaneous one because the drug is more bioavailable and higher plasma levels are attained after IM administration. The bioavailabilty of acepromazine after oral administration seems to be very poor and the plasma levels seem to be very low and erratic most probably due to the very high first pass effect. Thus, acepromazine should only have limited use or value when given orally.

APPENDIX

TABLE A-1:   Physical History of the Cats Used in the
               Pharmacokinetic Studies:

CAT ID	WEIGHT (Kg)	AGE (MONTHS)	SEX	TYPE[a]
RED1	4.8	22	MALE	DSH
GREEN1	3.7	25	MALE	DSH
GREEN2	3.7	24	MALE	DSH
RED2	5.1	21	MALE	DSH
MEAN	4.3	23		
SD[b]	0.73	1.83		

[a]DSH=domestic short haired.   [b] SD= standard deviation.

Table A-2

Medical History of the Horses Used in the Pharmacokinetic-Pharmacodynamic Studies

HORSE	AGE(YEARS)	SEX	WEIGHT(lbs)
RAISINa	–	male	1120
LETREMb	2	male	944
JUANITAc	8	female	1194
SARAd	13	female	1012
DAPPLERe	20	female	856
CHESTNUTf	15	female	856
MEAN	11.6	–	997
SD	6.87	–	139

a This horse was an adult gelding given acepromazine on 6/27/90 at a dose of 0.15 mg/kg and sampled through 24 hours. This horse was anesthetized at about 45 minutes post acepromazine administration. The anestheasia was thiobarbiturate, guaifenesin and halothane for about one hour.

b The study was performed on 12/4/89. It was an adult intact male horse referred for a heart condition. It had a vegetative lesion on the aortic valve with all clinical signs of regergitation. It showed no sign of heart failure. Post mortem results showed considerable congestive pulmonary problems secondary to the heart failure. Its blood gases (high pCO_2) confirmed it had a significant effect on ventilation.

c Juanita was an 8 year old mare with chronic forelamness used as a blood donor for the college of veterinary medicine.

d Sara was a blood donor at the college of veteraniry medicine

e Dappler had a sway back with colic when late in pregnancy

f Chestnut was in good health but required a special digestable diet.

TABLE A-3: Summary of the Plasma Concentration (ng/ml) vs time (min) Following IV Administration of 0.15 mg/kg Acepromazine Maleate to the Horse.

TIME	LETREN	JUANITA	CHESTNUT	SARA	DAPPLER	RAISIN
1	-	135.45	131.02	149.17	10.09	300
2	185.35	109.77	205.25	184.57	33.45	.193
3	105.57	132.15	116.77	85.02	64.74	133
4.5	61.03	91.230	79.93	42.95	34.54	85
6	52	81.59	-	-	30.25	-
7.5	45.85	47.11	41.5	61.49	20.96	72.4
10	45.5	46.33	50.94	20.33	21.37	90.8
12	40.4	40.57	-	27.76	21	-
14	33.32	30.51	34.14	-	4.08	-
15	-	-	-	-	-	64.8
18	37	27.81	42.58	26.21	105.75	-
20	30.13	22.76	31.16	-	4.55	60.7
25	28.05	19.72	29.95	-	-	-
30	26	16.6	-	28.05	-	48.7
40	21.38	22.66	26.33	4.73	6.37	59
45	-	-	-	-	-	-
50	23.43	12.19	-	11	22.82	-
55	-	-	-	-	-	37.3
60	22.2	7.15	18.88	5.48	11.36	30.9
70	-	-	-	-	-	38.1
75	24.05	-	27.32	-	-	-
85	-	-	-	-	-	36.8
90	23.96	-	18.81	-	-	-
95	-	-	-	-	-	29.7
100	-	-	-	-	-	-
106	-	-	-	-	-	-
120	-	-	22.04	-	-	28.2
180	-	-	14.95	-	-	-

TABLE A-4: Summary of the Blood Pressure (mm Hg) vs Time (min) After IV Administration of a 0.15 mg/kg dose of Acepromazine Maleate in the Horse.

TIME	SARA SP[a]	SARA DP[b]	SARA MP[c]	JUANITA SP	JUANITA DP	JUANITA MP	DAPPLER SP	DAPPLER DP	DAPPLER MP	CHESTNUT SP	CHESTNUT DP	CHESTNUT MP	LETREN SP	LETREN DP	LETREN MP
0	141	121	134	124	65	86	188	81	118	144	71	107	138	42	89
1	141	85	116	122	54	87	-	-	-	41	75	105	132	47	81
2	176	97	125	100	56	77	122	83	103	149	82	100	136	43	78
3	159	82	106	114	59	80	120	94	108	136	76	97	138	43	79
4.5	155	101	80	104	59	79	136	73	93	137	79	99	133	49	83
6	148	79	104	99	55	72	130	70	88	139	86	109	132	42	77
7.5	158	77	101	99	57	72	132	65	88	135	78	95	125	44	76
10	116	61	89	96	58	74	129	66	85	119	65	84	147	39	72
12	125	63	83	112	58	75	116	66	82	126	70	86	150	34	75
14	126	53	85	108	57	72	122	61	79	116	63	79	165	39	79
16	-	-	-	95	58	73	111	58	77	112	64	79	133	30	67
18	112	54	73	105	56	72	113	55	73	112	67	81	144	36	69
20	122	62	80	100	63	74	113	60	76	111	61	76	124	22	67
25	123	62	79	110	50	75	109	55	71	116	63	90	130	38	71
30	128	63	81	105	55	70	96	58	72	99	51	67	144	40	72
40	111	60	76	91	57	69	98	57	68	103	56	70	140	35	70
50	114	65	77	108	56	70	91	56	68	107	61	74	131	47	68
60	118	63	76	100	57	76	102	56	69	97	58	72	143	42	74
75	100	64	61	114	40	63	98	31	70	94	58	69	112	37	74
90	109	69	84	105	55	68	100	58	72	98	66	77	137	44	74
120	110	71	85	78	37	85	101	56	77	103	64	75	128	37	73
150	114	65	75	82	55	73	112	84	72	95	63	72	95	63	72
180	102	62	84	93	48	66	-	-	-	101	61	76	101	61	76
210	107	80	71	111	61	78	112	68	83	107	62	75	107	62	75
240	122	74	91	142	87	10	109	68	79	109	67	79	109	67	79

[a]Systolic blood pressure. [b]Diastolic blood pressure. [c]Mean blood pressure.

TABLE A-5:   Heart Rate As A Function of Time After
an IV Administration of 0.15 mg/kg Dose
of Acepromazine For The Horses of Interest.

TIME	SARA	JUANITA	DAPPLER	CHESTNUT	LEIREN
1	42	43	43	41	58
2	.43	44	43	32	53
3	49	44	40	34	53
4.5	40	46	37	32	42
6	41	54	38	34	52
7.5	45	47	38	33	53
10	113	56	39	31	53
12	46	38	37	35	52
14	48	38	42	35	52
16	-	36	46	37	48
18	37	45	47	37	52
20	37	36	46	40	53
25	33	45	62	47	51
30	35	33	51	48	52
40	33	41	56	33	50
50	30	31	53	32	53
60	32	45	34	30	52
75	28	40	34	30	52
90	35	32	49	30	49
120	32	30	41	28	50
150	34	28	32	32	54
180	47	36	-	31	49
210	40	33	37	29	51
240	40	36	40	36	50

TABLE A-6A: Summary of the Sedative and CNS Effects as a Function of Time for the Horse of Interest After an IV Administration of a 0.15 mg/kg of Acepromazine Maleate.

TIME	SARA MVT[a]	NR[b]	PPR[c]	HC[d]	ELD[e]	JUANITA MVT	NR	PPR	HC	ELD	DAPPER MVT	NR	PPR	HC	ELD
0	1	1	1	1	1	1	1	1	1	1	1	1	1	1	1
2	1.5	1	1	1	1	1	1	1	1	1	1	1	1	1	1
3	1.5	1	1	1.5	1.5	1.5	1	1	1	1	2	1	1	2	2
4.5	2	1	1	3	1.5	1.5	1	1	1.5	1	2	1	1	2	2
6	2.5	1	1.5	3	1.5	2	1	1	2	2	2	1	1	2	2
7.5	3	2	1.5	4	1.5	2	1	1	3	2	2	1	1	3	2
10	3	2.5	1.5	4	2	3	2	1	3	3	1	1	1	3	3
12	3	2.5	1.5	4	2.5	3	1	2	3	3	3	2	1	3	3
14	3	2.5	2	3	2.5	3	1	1	4	3	3	1	3	3	3
16	3	2.5	2	3	2.5	3	1	1	4	3	3	1	3	3	3
18	3	2.5	2	3	2.5	2	1	1	4	3	3.5	1	2	3	3
20	2.5	2	2	3	2.5	2	1	1	3	3	3	1	2	3	3
25	2.5	2	2.5	3	2.5	2.5	1	1	2	2	3	1	2	4	2
30	3	1	1	3	2.5	2.5	1	1	2	2	2.5	1	1	3	2
40	3	1	1	4	2.5	2	1	1	2	2	2.5	1	1	2	2
50	3	1	1	3.5	2.5	2	1	1	2	2	2	1	1	2	2
60	3	1	1	3.5	2.5	2	1	1	2	2	2	1	1	2	2
75	3	1	1	0	2.5	2	1	1	2	2	2	1	1	2	2
90	3	1	1	3	2.5	2	1	1	2	2.5	2	1	1	2	2
120	2.5	1	1	3	2	2	1	1	2	1.5	2	1	1	2	2
150	2	1	1	2	1.5	1	1	1	1.5	1.5	2	1	1	2	2
180	1.5	1	1	2	1.5	1.5	1	1	2.5	1.5	1.5	1	1	1	1.5
210	1.5	1	1	2	1	2	1	1	1	1	1.5	1	1	1.5	1.5
240	1.5	1	1	1	1	2	1	1	1	1	1	1	1	1	1

[a] Movement
[b] Reaction to noise
[c] Pinprick reaction
[d] Head carriage
[e] Eyelid droop

TABLE A-6B: Summary of the Sedative and CNS Effects as a Function of Time for Horse of Interest After an IV Administration of 0.15 mg/kg Dose of Acepromazine Maleate

TIME	MT	NB	FER	HC	ELD	MT	NB	FER	HC	ELD
0	1	1	1	1	1	1	1	1	1	1
2	1.5	1	1.5	1.5	1	1	1	1	1	1
3	1.5	1	1.2	1.5	1	1	1	1	1	1
4.5	1.5	1	1.5	1.5	1	2	1	1	1	2
6	2	1	1.5	2	2	2	1	1	2	2
7.5	2	1	1.5	2	2	2	1	1	2	1
10	1	2	2	2	2.5	2.5	1	3	2.5	
12	2	1	2	2	2	2.5	2	1	3	2.5
14	2	1	2	2	2	2.5	2	1	4	2.5
16	2	1	2	2	2	2	1	1	3	2.5
18	2	1	2	2.5	2	2	1	1	2.5	2
20	2.5	1	2	3	2	2	1	1	2	2.5
25	2.5	1	2	3	2	2	1	1	3	2.5
30	3	1	2	3	2	2	1	1	3	2.5
40	3	1	2	2.5	3	1.5	1	0	3	
50	1	1.5	3	3	1	1	A	A	2.5	
60	3	1	1.5	2.5	3	1.5	A	A	2	
75	2	2.5	1	1	2.5	2	1	1	A	2
90	2.5	1	1	2.5	1.5	1	1	1	1	1
120	2	1	1	1.5	1	1	1	1	1	1
150	1.5	1	1	1.5	1	1	1	1	1	1.5
180	1.5	1	1	1.5	1	1	1	1	2.5	2
210	1.5	1	1	1	1	1	1	1	1	1
240	1.5	1	1	1	1	1	1	1	1	1

TABLE A-7: Blood Gases vs Time After IV Administration of a 0.15 mg/kg Dose of Acepromazine in the Horse.

TIME	SARA				JUANITA				DAPPLER				CHESTNUT				LEMON			
	pH	PCO_2	PO_2	B	pH	PCO_2	PO_2	B	pH	PCO_2	PO_2	B	pH	PCO_2	PO_2	B	pH	PCO_2	PO_2	B
0	7.39	42.7	86	0.7	7.45	42.8	98	5.7	7.4	43.5	113	2.4	7.37	40.5	125	-1.9	7.4	43.5	123	2.4
1	-	-	-	-	-	-	-	-	-	-	-	-	7.42	38.1	117	0.2	-	-	-	-
2	-	-	-	-	-	-	-	-	-	-	-	-	7.43	35.8	85	-0.5	-	-	-	-
3	7.38	41.2	104	-0.4	7.48	38.9	83	6	7.43	41.9	111	3.3	7.43	35.8	85	-0.5	7.43	41.9	111	3.3
6	7.39	40.4	90	-0.7	7.48	40.3	77	6.7	7.44	40.8	105	4.1	7.36	39.4	110	-3.1	7.45	40.8	105	4.1
10	7.42	37.1	110	-0.1	7.43	45.2	84	6.1	7.43	41.9	122	3.4	7.37	40.6	104	-1.9	7.43	41.9	122	3.4
16	7.39	40.6	94	0	7.42	44.4	85	4.8	7.47	37.2	78	3.6	7.34	44.3	107	-1.9	7.47	37.2	78	3.6
20	7.4	38	101	-0.9	7.41	45.7	87	4.6	7.42	42	113	2.8	7.36	40.6	107	-2.7	7.42	42	113	2.8
25	7.38	40.2	100	-1	7.38	49.2	88	4.3	7.46	37.7	95	2.9	7.34	43.4	105	-2.5	7.46	37.7	95	2.9
30	7.37	42.6	101	-0.4	7.4	46.7	86	4.5	7.47	38.1	94	4	7.34	40.9	104	-2.6	7.47	38.1	94	4
40	7.39	40.7	98	0.1	7.41	45.5	96	4.3	7.46	38.6	80	3.4	7.35	41.3	118	-1.5	7.46	38.6	80	3.4
50	7.39	41.1	101	0.4	7.42	44.6	94	4.2	7.4	44.2	102	2.3	7.35	43.4	112	-2.3	7.4	44.2	102	2.3
60	7.36	44.8	101	-0.2	7.43	44.7	88	5.4	7.43	39.9	105	2.1	7.33	43.4	112	-2.3	7.43	39.9	105	2.1
75	7.4	40.9	132	0.7	7.42	44.2	94	4.7	7.36	45.4	120	0.5	7.57	42.3	104	-2.3	7.36	45.4	120	0.5
90	7.39	41.8	94	0.8	7.43	46.3	106	4.8	7.45	39.2	78	3.3	7.35	41.9	109	-3	7.45	39.2	78	3.3
120	7.38	42.2	94	0	7.45	40.1	100	4.1	7.39	44.3	114	1.9	7.33	42.9	103	-2.3	7.39	44.3	114	1.9
150	7.39	42.2	97	0.4	7.45	42.6	101	5.7	7.4	43.1	114	2.1	7.37	39	116	-3.7	7.4	43.1	114	2.1
180	7.4	44	114	2.3	7.41	42.8	109	2.4	7.39	42.3	112	0.7	7.35	32.7	118	-3.7	7.39	42.3	112	0.7
210	7.38	41.2	93	-0.3	7.4	44.9	107	3.1	7.39	39.7	125	-0.7	7.32	42.6	95	-3.8	7.39	39.7	125	-0.7
240	7.37	44.4	92	0.7	7.42	43.3	100	3.4	7.42	40.9	102	2.2	7.33	41	101	-4.2	7.42	40.9	102	2.2

TABLE A-8: Hematocrit vs Time (min) After an IV Administration of 0.15 mg/kg of Acepromazine Maleate to the Horse.

TIME	SARA	JUANITA	DAPPLER	CHESTNUT	LEIREN
1	33	36	40	36	40
2	34	38	35	36	40
3	29	38	36	34	40
4.5	33	36	36	34	40
6	32	35	35	33	40
7.5	32	35	34	34	40
10	29	32	34	33	40
12	28	32	33	32	39
14	28	30	32	32	39
16	29	31	32	32	38
18	29	31	32	32	39
20	28	32	31	31	36
25	28	31	32	31	38
30	24	30	32	30	36
40	26	-	32	31	36
50	28	28	30	29	37
60	26	28	29	30	37
75	27	-	29	30	36
90	27	29	28	30	35
120	27	30	27	-	36
150	26	30	28	30	37
180	25	30	28	30	37
210	26	30	28	31	31
240	27	23	28	-	31

TABLE A-9:   Plasma Concentration (ng/ml) vs Time (min) After IV Administration of 0.3 mg/kg Dose of Acepromazine To Four Cats.

TIME	CAT1 GREEN	CAT1 RED	CAT2 Green	CAT2 RED
1	-	-	110	-
1.5	405	322	-	591
2.5	-	-	94	277
3	315	182	-	-
3.6	-	-	-	206
4	-	-	86	-
4.5	443	-	-	-
5	-	-	-	151
6	189	151	78	-
7.5	172	126	-	169
8	-	-	-	124
9	185	134	-	-
10	-	-	55	92
12.5	146	114	-	-
13	-	-	55	92
15	187	100	-	-
18.5	210	127	-	-
20	-	-	-	123
24	189	95	-	-
26	-	-	52	-
30	132	114	60	-
41	-	-	31	-
44	-	83	-	-
45	-	-	-	54
46	70	-	-	-
50	-	-	28	-
60	66	-	26	-
89	50	-	17	-
93	-	56	-	-
118	-	-	10	-
121	-	61	-	-
129	16	-	-	-
150	-	48	15	-
180	-	61	-	-
210	8	28	65	-
240	-	27	-	-

TABLE A-10:   Plasma Concentration (ng/ml) as a Function of Time (min) After an Oral administration of 10 mg Tablet of Acepromazine Maleate to Four Cats.

TIME	CAT1 GREEN	CAT1 RED	CAT2 GREEN	CAT2 RED
35	–	51	–	0
40	–	–	68	0
45	–	37	–	0
50	–	–	66	0
60	51	56	93	0
70	–	–	75	0
80	–	–	60	0
90	60	71	83	0
110	–	–	53	0
120	107	81	–	0
150	250	–	–	0
155	–	–	33	0
170	–	–	59	0
180	242	57	–	0
210	122	48	–	0
240	71	27	27	0
300	66	–	–	0
360	62	–	–	0

TABLE A-11: Plasma Concentration (ng/ml) as a Function of Time (min) After Subcutaneous Administration of 0.3 mg/kg of Acepromazine Maleate to Four Cats.

TIME	CAT1 GREEN	CAT1 RED	CAT2 GREEN	CAT2 RED
4	29	-	45	-
8	34	-	-	13
12	40	56	43	17
16	46	-	44	4
19	-	36	-	9
20	45	-	56	21
23	-	19	47	-
27	-	28	63	29
29	27	-	67	-
31	-	23	-	-
35	28	21	-	22
40	24	-	52	19
50	27	66	54	14
60	18	-	47	38
75	-	46	48	31
90	17	22	-	22
120	-	24	43	34
150	-	17	32	6
210	-	25	-	38
240	-	-	-	28
300	-	16	-	-

TABLE A-12: Plasma concentration (ng/ml) as a Function of Time (min) After an Intramuscular Administration of a 0.3 mg/kg of Acepromazine Maleat to Four Cats.

TIME	CAT1 GREEN	CAT1 RED	CAT2 GREEN	CAT2 RED
4	-	-	NA	44
8	-	11	NA	36
9	35.2	-	NA	-
12	-	213	NA	63
16	130	293	NA	77
20	312	312	NA	65
23	-	396	NA	-
25	200	-	NA	164
30	133	133	NA	48
40	110	-	NA	38
50	73	-	NA	24
60	61	-	NA	-
75	57	176	NA	-
120	24	-	NA	-
150	-	-	NA	22
200	-	46	NA	-
210	-	-	NA	10
240	-	-	NA	24
300	-	-	NA	21

TABLE A-13: Summary of the Hematocrit as a Function of Time (min) For All Routes of Administration of Acepromazine Maleate in the Cat.

TIME	CAT GREEN1				CAT RED1				CAT GREEN2				CAT RED2			
	IV	PO	IM	SC	IV	PO	SC	IM	IV	PO	SC	IV	PO	SC	IM	
0	35	34	20	28	29	34	36	31	34	32	30	39	32	31	31	
1	-	-	-	-	33	-	-	-	34	-	-	40	-	-	-	
1.5	30	30	-	-	-	-	-	-	-	-	-	39	31	-	-	
2	-	-	-	26	33	30	35	30	32	32	-	37	-	-	30	
2.5	34	29	27	-	-	-	-	-	31	-	-	34	31	33	-	
3.5	-	-	-	-	-	-	-	-	31	-	25	-	-	-	-	
4	33	28	28	28	30	32	32	30	30	32	-	35	29	30	28	
4.5	-	-	-	-	-	-	-	-	-	30	24	34	30	-	-	
5.5	30	29	28	23	29	-	32	29	30	29	28	30	30	24	28	
6	30	27	28	28	27	31	31	28	26	-	28	29	30	28	28	
7.5	32	25	26	24	27	30	31	28	27	29	25	28	26	27	27	
8	-	-	-	22	-	30	28	28	27	28	23	28	26	26	-	
9	29	25	28	23	24	29	28	-	29	27	23	26	-	-	24	
10	-	-	-	24	25	29	25	27	-	24	27	25	-	28	28	
12	25	22	27	24	24	28	25	27	29	23	27	22	24	25	27	
14	-	-	-	22	-	28	23	26	29	30	24	24	24	24	24	
15	29	23	23	21	22	25	20	24	28	29	24	26	21	25	26	
16	24	21	25	20	14	24	20	22	-	28	23	26	24	25	-	
18	22	21	26	20	20	25	21	23	31	24	-	-	20	22	27	
20	23	20	26	19	22	21	21	23	30	23	24	24	20	23	22	
23	24	21	23	20	19	22	22	23	30	28	23	23	17	21	27	
25	27	21	23	21	-	21	21	23	23	22	21	20	17	19	22	
26	20	22	23	20	25	20	18	23	26	25	22	20	19	20	18	
29	-	-	-	-	-	-	-	-	-	-	23	-	18	-	19	
30	22	21	25	20	-	21	20	-	24	-	-	21	17	20	20	
360	26	21	27	21	-	-	-	22	23	-	22	21	-	20	19	

Table A-14: Rating scale for the CNS and sedative effects

RATING SCALE

Horse I.D.:

Date:

Time:

Please rate the following five characteristics of the horse at this time on the five point scales provided. Please circle the appropriate numbers.

A. Movement / Proprioception   0   1   2   3   4

---

         4. No movement at all (collapsed or ready to collapse)
         3. Very lethargic
         2. Slightly affected
         1. Normal for environment
         0. More than normal activity for environment

B. Reaction to noise   0   1   2 . 3   4

---

         4. None
         3. Markedly affected
         2. Slightly affected
         1. Normal reaction
         0. Excessive reaction

C. Reaction to pin prick   0   1   2   3   4

---

         4. None
         3. Markedly affected
         2. Slightly affected
         1. Normal reaction
         0. Excessive reaction

D. Head carriage   0   1   2   3   4

---

    4. Down

    3. Horizontal

    2. Slight effect

    1. Normal

    0. Excessive movement / elevation

E. Eyelid droop   0   1   2   3   4

---

    4. Closed
    3. 50% or more closed
    2. Slight effect
    1. Normal
    0. Excessively wide-eyed

BIBLIOGRAPHY

(1)- R. Byck in " The Pharmacological Basis of Therapeutics", L. S. Goodman and A. Gilman, Eds., Macmillan Publishing Co., Inc., New York, Chapter 12, 1975.

(2)- P. Charpentier, P. Gaillot, J. Gaudelin, C.R. Hebd seanc. Academie Science, Paris 232: 2232-2233. 1951

(3)- S. Courvoisier, J. Fournel, R. Ducrot, M. Kolsky and P. Koetshet, Arch. Int. Pharmacodynamyc. 92:305. 1953

(4)-H. Laborit, P. Huguenard and R. Alluane, Presse Med, 60:206. 1952.

(5)- H. Lehman and G. Hanrahan, A.M.A. Archs Neurol. Psychiatry, 71:227. 1954.

(6)- Dr. E. krimmer pharmacology handouts for the pharmacology 1 class, University of Pittsburgh. 1984.

(7)- A. Carlson and M. Lindquist, Acta Pharmacol Toxicol 20:140 1963

(8)-Veterinary Pharmaceuticals and Biologicals, sixth edition, Veterinary Medium Publishing Company, p 858, Lenexa, Kansas 1989.

(9)- B. Parry, G. Anderson and C. Gay, Aust Vet J, 59:148-151. 1982.

(10)-W. Muir, R. Skarda and W. Sheehan. Am J Vet Res 40:1518 1979.

(11)-W. Muir and R. Hamlin. Am J Vet Res 36:1439-1442. 1975

(12)-B. Parry and G. Anderson. J Vet Pharmacol Therap 6:121-126 1983.

(13)-N. Popovic, F. Mullane and O Yhap, Am J Vet Res. 33:1819.

(14)-B. Coulter, S. Whelan, R. Wilson et al, Cornel Vet 71:76 1981.

(14)-B. Coulter, S. Whelan, R. Wilson et al, <u>Cornel Vet</u> 71:76 1981.

(15)-H. Dodman, D. Seeler, M. Court, <u>Br Vet J</u> 140:505 1984.

(16)-G. Mackenzie and D. Snow, <u>Vet Rec.</u> 101:30.

(17)-C. Frank, <u>Vet Rec</u>, 87:497 1970.

(18)-P. Miller, I. Martin, J. Kohnke and R. Rose, <u>Research in Veterinary Science</u>. 42:318-325. 1987.

(19)- J. Garland and K. White, <u>Vet Rec</u> 83:641 1966.

(20)-K. White, <u>Vet Rec</u> 83:688 1968.

(21)-A. Waechter, <u>J Am Vet Med Assoc</u> 180:73 1982.

(22)-H. Pearson and B. Weaver, <u>Equine vet J</u> 10:85 1978.

(23)-A. Becket, M. Beaven and A. Robinson, <u>Biochem Pharmacol</u> 12:779 1963.

(24)-E. Usdin, <u>Crit. Rev. Clin. Lab. Sci</u> 2:347 1971.

(25)-I. Forest and D. Green. <u>J Forensic Science</u> 17:592 1972.

(26)-J. Craig, <u>First Int. Symp. Psychopharmacol Serv. Cent. Bull</u>, 2:44. 1962.

(27)-S. Curry in " Antipsychotics", Burrows, Norman and Davies Editors. Chapter 7 pp 79-97. Elseviers Science Publishers, New York, N.Y. 1983.

(28)-E. Essien, D. Lowan and A. Beckett, <u>J Pharm. Pharmacol</u> 27:334 1975.

(29)-J. Buckley, M. Steenberg, H. Berry and A. Manian in "Phenothiazines and structurally related drugs", I. Forrest, C. Carr and E. Usdin Eds., Raven Press, New York pp 617-631 1974.

(30)-E. Dewey, G. Maylin, J. Ebel and J. Herion, <u>Drug Met and Disp</u> vol 9 #1 pp30-36 1981.

(31)-S. Dahl and R. Strandjord, Clin. Pharmacol. Therap. 21:437 1976.

(32)-L. Whitfield, P. Kaul and M. Clark, J Pharmacokin. Biopharm. 6:187 1980.

(33)-J. Loo, K. Midha and I. McGilveray, Comm. in Psychopharmacol. 4:121, 1980.

(34)- J. Maxwell, M. Carrella, J. Parke, R. Williams, G. Mould and S. Curry, Clin. Sci 43:143. 1977.

(35)-S. Curry, Br. J. Clin. Pharmacol. 3:20-8. 1976.

(36)-S. Curry in "Plasma levels of psychotropic drugs and clinical response." G. Burnes and T. Nauer Eds. Marcel Dekker, New York, N.Y. 1981.

(37)-S..Stavchansky, J. Wallace, R. Geary, G. Hecht, C. Robb and P. Wu. J Pharm Science. 76:6 pp441-445 1987.

(38)-R. Casper, D.Garver, H. Dekirmenjian, S. Chang and J. Davis, Arch. Gen. Psychiatry 37: 301-305.

(39)-N. Svenson, C. Olofsson, U. Axelsson and R. Mantenson. Ther drug Monit 9:426-432 1987.

(40)-P. Sundaresan and L. Rivera- Calimlim, J. Pharmacol. Exp. Ther. 194:593 1975.

(41)-S. Curry, J. Pharm. Pharmacol, 22:193. 1970.

(42)-S. Ballard, T. Shultz, A. Kownack, W. Blake and T. Tobin, J. vet. Pharm. Ther. 5:21-31. 1982.

(43)-S. Curry and B. Brodie, Fed Proc. 26:761. 1967.

(44)-S. Curry, Anal. Chem, 40:1251. 1968.

(45)-S. Ballard, T. Tobin, J of Toxicol and Env Health. 7:745-751. 1981.

(46)-D. Courtot, Bul. Soc. Sci. Vet et med compare, 76:5 pp361-366. 1974.

(47)-P. Hinderling, J. Bres, and E. Garrett, J. Pharm Sci,

BIOGRAPHICAL SKETCH

Patrick John Marroum, who is of Palestinian descent, was born August 9, 1960, in Beirut, Lebanon. He attended the College De LaSalle in Beirut until the middle school. Due to the civil war in Lebanon he transferred to the College Protestant Francais where he finished high school and obtained both the French and Lebanese scientific baccalaureat degrees. In 1980 he completed all the pre-pharmacy courses at the Beirut University College.

In 1984, he earned a Bachelor in Pharmacy (Magna Cum Laude) from the University of Pittsburgh.

Mr. Marroum began his graduate education at the University of Florida in 1984 under the supervision of Dr. Edward R. Garrett. Due to the failing health of Dr. Garrett, he transferred to Dr. Stephen Curry. He pursued his work towards the Ph.D. degree with a major in pharmacy. During this period, he was the President of the Table Tennis Club and the Arab Cultural Club at the University of Florida. He also was a member of the Pharmacy Student Council as the graduate student representative.

He will be employed by the United States Food and Drug Administration as a reviewer for New Drug Applications.

I certify that I have read this study and that in my opinion it conforms to acceptable standards of scholarly presentation and is fully adequate, in scope and quality, as a dissertation for the degree of Doctor of Philosophy.

_____
Dr. Stephen H. Curry, Chairman
Professor of Pharmaceutics

I certify that I have read this study and that in my opinion it conforms to acceptable standards of scholarly presentation and is fully adequate, in scope and quality, as a dissertation for the degree of Doctor of Philosophy.

_____
Dr. Edward R. Garrett
Graduate Research Professor
Emeritus of Pharmaceutics

I certify that I have read this study and that in my opinion it conforms to acceptable standards of scholarly presentation and is fully adequate, in scope and quality, as a dissertation for the degree of Doctor of Philosophy.

_____
Dr. Hartmut Derendorf
Associate Professor
of Pharmaceutics

I certify that I have read this study and that in my opinion it conforms to acceptable standards of scholarly presentation and is fully adequate, in scope and quality, as a dissertation for the degree of Doctor of Philosophy.

Dr. Stephen G. Schulman
Professor of Pharmaceutics

I certify that I have read this study and that in my opinion it conforms to acceptable standards of scholarly presentation and is fully adequate, in scope and quality, as a dissertation for the degree of Doctor of Philosophy.

Dr. Alistair Webb
Associate Professor
of Veterinary Medicine

I certify that I have read this study and that in my opinion it conforms to acceptable standards of scholarly presentation and is fully adequate, in scope and quality, as a dissertation for the degree of Doctor of Philosophy.

Dr. Willis Person
Professor of Chemistry

This dissertation was submitted to the Graduate Faculty of the College of Pharmacy and to the Graduate School and was accepted as partial fulfillment of the requirements for the degree of Doctor of Philosophy.

August 1990

Dean, College of Pharmacy

Dean, Graduate School